Shed Ten Years in Ten Weeks

JULIAN WHITAKER, M.D.
and CAROL COLMAN

SIMON & SCHUSTER

SIMON & SCHUSTER
Rockefeller Center
1230 Avenue of the Americas
New York, NY 10020

SIMON & SCHUSTER and colophon are registered trademarks of
Simon & Schuster Inc.

Designed by Irving Perkins Associates

Manufactured in the United States of America

7   9   10   8   6

Library of Congress Cataloging-in-Publication Data
Whitaker, Julian M.
Shed ten years in ten weeks / Julian Whitaker, and Carol Colman.
p.   cm.
Includes bibliographical references (p.   ) and index.
1. Rejuvenation. 2. Health. I. Colman, Carol. II. Title.
RA776.75.W48 1997
613—dc21   97-18381 CIP
ISBN 0-684-84478-8

Acknowledgments

We would like to thank the many people who helped to make this book a reality. Much thanks to Laurie Bernstein, who believed in this project from the start, and who helped mold and shape the book from its inception. We also owe a debt of gratitude to Annie O'Connor for her vision and hard work and to Michele Martin for her guidance and keen insight. Thanks also to Ted Landry who has worked long hours to expedite this project.

In addition, a very special thanks to Peggy Dace for her intelligence and efficiency.

Thanks also to Marge Hoffman, who helped to coordinate everyone's busy schedules with skill and grace.

Much thanks to Daren Gregson, Ph.D., and Idel Kelly for their special contributions.

Dr. Whitaker would like to thank his agent, Laura Blake Peterson, for her support.

Carol Colman would like to thank her agent, Richard Curtis, for helping her every step along the way. In addition, she would like to thank her husband, Michael Gerber, and her son, Josh Gerber, for their patience, love, and encouragement.

I dedicate this book to readers who will use it to improve their health and enrich their lives.

Julian Whitaker, M.D.

Contents

Contents

Introduction

∅

The Ten Simple Steps to Age Loss

Take out your calendar. Count ten weeks from today. Circle that date. I will make you a promise: On that date you will look and feel a full ten years younger if you follow my ten-step Age Loss Program. It will not be magic, nor will it be your imagination playing tricks on you. In exactly ten weeks from today you will actually feel stronger, sexier, and sharper. You will feel renewed and *be* renewed, and ready to take on the world. Sound too good to be true? It's not.

The promise of *Shed Ten Years in Ten Weeks* is a profoundly simple one: With the right intervention, a decade's worth of age-related damage can be reversed in ten weeks' time. *Shed Ten Years in Ten Weeks* will show you how to turn back the clock to a time when you felt stronger, more in control, healthier, and more vigorous; to a time when you looked terrific and functioned at your mental, physical, and sexual peak.

This unique and simple ten-step program is based on twenty years of experience with thousands of patients. Thousands of different men and women of all ages have come to the Whitaker Wellness Institute in Newport Beach, California, and have left feeling and acting mentally and physically "younger." When I say younger, I mean that their bodies became stronger and leaner, and had improved muscle mass and tone. Their skin looked markedly refreshed. Their brains functioned better. Their sex lives were enhanced.

These stunning and palpable improvements are only the external signs, however, of what is going on inside their bodies. Experience has taught me that we have to take care of ourselves from the outside in as well as from the inside out. In other words, we need to take care of our internal health as well as our physical appearance, and our mental and spiritual well-being. You may think I'm stating the obvious, but I think the reason so many programs fail is that they focus on one body part at a time instead of treating the whole person. What happens to one part of the body can profoundly affect another part.

Shed Ten Years in Ten Weeks is comprehensive and easy to follow. Each step contains specific information on what you need to do and exactly how to do it. Best of all, you will find the Age Loss Program an enjoyable, life-affirming experience.

Before I tell you more about the Age Loss Program and teach you the ten easy steps, let me tell you a little bit about me and my medical practice.

I come from a medical family. My father is a prominent surgeon in Atlanta, Georgia, and one of the most skillful and compassionate surgeons I have ever known. My older brother is a radiologist in Atlanta and highly respected in his field. It is no surprise, therefore, that from the age of ten I have wanted to be a doctor. I received my undergraduate degree from Dartmouth College, and I entered Emory University Medical School in 1966.

I did my medical-surgical internship at Grady Memorial Hospital in Atlanta, an extremely busy teaching hospital, and following my internship I began an orthopedic surgery residency at the University of California in San Francisco. It was there that I began to question the medical profession and my place in it. It bothered me that surgeons seemed to derive their greatest personal satisfaction from the drama of surgery itself rather than from relating to and working with patients. I felt there was something dreadfully wrong with the medical profession's narrow focus on surgery, drugs, and other risky procedures rather than taking a more natural, healing approach.

At about this time I began working in the emergency room of a hospital in southern California, and it was here that a patient inadvertently helped me find my calling. A thirty-four-year-old woman came in for treatment of a sprained ankle. Her ankle was swollen, but she was the picture of health. Her eyes sparkled, her skin glowed, and she was slim and muscular. She looked completely out of place in the hospital. As I bandaged her ankle, I asked her how she stayed so fit, and she told me that she simply took a lot of vitamins and minerals, exercised regularly, and ate a healthy diet.

As we talked, it dawned on me that she was the first healthy patient that I had examined in years. And ironically, the things that she was doing to keep herself healthy were the very things that I had *not* been taught in medical school. Suddenly I realized that the answer was all around me: We doctors tend to spend all our time looking at and studying *illness*. We focus so narrowly on how to cure patients after they get sick that we do not concentrate on how to overtake illness before it overtakes the body. From that moment on I knew that I wanted to practice a different kind of medicine and be a different kind of doctor. I knew that I did not want merely to treat patients who had already succumbed to disease. I wanted my practice to be devoted to maximizing my patients' health and keeping them healthy. But first I needed to do more research to fill the gaps in my education.

I went to work for Dr. William Currier, a physician in Pasadena, California, who had given up a career in ear, nose, and throat surgery to specialize in nutrition and preventive medicine. Since I had learned so little about nutrition in medical school, I was particularly intrigued by Dr. Currier's practice. He was one of the earliest supporters of Dr. Nathan Pritikin, a little-known inventor regarded in the 1970s as "radical" for proposing low-fat nutrition as a therapy for heart disease, diabetes, and high blood pressure. With Dr. Currier's guidance I studied Dr. Pritikin's early monographs on diabetes. Numerous scientific articles published in the 1920s and 1930s demonstrated that diet could be used to treat diabetes and even eliminate the need for insulin therapy in some patients, yet I had not even heard about them in medical school. (And I'm sad to report that medical students today are still not being taught any more nutrition than I was.)

I visited the Pritikin Longevity Center and in 1976 joined the staff—a critical turning point in my career and in my professional point of view. For the first time I actually understood what it meant to make a patient well.

At Pritikin I saw desperately ill people suffering from advanced heart disease who were literally brought back to life, and not through dangerous drugs or risky surgical procedures but through diet and exercise. The difference between what I saw at Pritikin and at the hospitals where I had trained was shocking. I had admitted and discharged hundreds of patients, and although many of them had improved, none had actually gotten well. I remember seeing heart patients leave the hospital laden with prescriptions, only to return for surgery and other treatment, sometimes over and over again. But at Pritikin I did not experience this revolving door effect. I saw patients actually cured and given back their lives. I saw diabetics throw away their insulin. I saw patients lower their blood pressure enough to get off medication. I saw angina disappear.

14

I realized that Pritikin's approach was so successful because he did not just treat symptoms of disease, he treated the underlying cause of disease: poor diet and an unhealthy lifestyle. Once these patients made positive changes in their behavior, their bodies began to heal. This had a profound impact on me. I knew that I would devote the rest of my career to teaching patients how to make—and keep—themselves well.

I undertook the study of nutrition and lesser known but very effective remedies for many medical conditions, such as vitamins, minerals, and herbs. In the process I developed my own unique style of medical practice, which I have employed for more than two decades at the Whitaker Wellness Institute. Here my staff and I have treated more than fifteen thousand patients who have come to us from around the world. Most of these patients travel to the institute to undergo a rigorous week-long evaluation and treatment regimen embracing every aspect of their physical and emotional health. Without leaving your home, you, too, can follow my program. But before you do, it is important for you to understand our philosophy.

At the Whitaker Wellness Institute we do not confine our treatment plan to "fixing" one ailment or repairing one organ system as is done in conventional medicine. The underlying philosophy of our treatment approach—and of the Age Loss Program—is twofold. First, we operate from the premise that all the systems of the body are interconnected and that a weakness in one will affect others. In other words, for the total body to function well, each part must work well independently and in concert. Second, we help people who are ill to improve their nutrition significantly, using a therapeutic formula of vitamins and minerals. Health is almost always dramatically improved.

Although I do prescribe conventional drug therapies and even recommend surgery when necessary, I routinely depart from conventional approaches and employ alternative remedies, especially a wide range of nutritional supplements. When I say "supplements," I am not talking about the sprinkling of vitamins and minerals in the Recommended Daily Allowances, nor am I talking about the meager ration of supplements found in most popular multivitamins. Rather, I am referring to my *Age Loss ODAs* (Optimal Daily Allowance), a whole new generation of sophisticated, high-tech supplements—vitamins, minerals, herbs, and essential fatty acids. Many of these are not yet known to the general public but have potent *anti*-aging and health-promoting properties. They are often more effective than prescription drugs and without the side effects. These side effects occur because drugs work *against* the bodily processes. In contrast, the supplements that I use get the job done by working in harmony with the body. I believe that the most effective therapies are not necessarily those that declare "war" on a particular ailment (and turn our body into a battleground) but those that fortify our body's own defense systems. These therapies give us the strength and stamina we need to repel or correct problems from within.

Accordingly, my Age Loss Program utilizes alternative therapies to renew the body by bolstering the same organ systems that are weakened by the aging process. Nearly all the supplements that I recommend in this book are sold over the counter at neighborhood pharmacies and health food stores. In some special circumstances I recommend that you consult your doctor about supplements that are available only by prescription.

Before you begin the Age Loss Program, you should be aware of the important rules that we live by at the Whitaker Wellness Institute:

1. It Is Never Too Late.

Although I preach the virtues of wellness, many of the patients who come to my clinic do so because they are profoundly ill. I see patients who have serious heart conditions, debilitating diseases, sky-high blood pressure, and who are obese. Many patients are so sick that they have lost all hope and are resigned to living out the rest of their lives as invalids. They are ready to quit their jobs and cut back on the activities they love. After following my program, their lives are changed for the better. Many are now running businesses, traveling around the world, and leading full, active, and healthy lives.

So remember that it is never too late, and you are never too old to do something positive for yourself. You are never too sick to reclaim your health and body. The Age Loss Program will show you how.

Don't get me wrong: I do not claim that the Age Loss Program can cure every ailment or turn an eighty-year-old into an eighteen-year-old. What I do know is that my Age Loss Program can profoundly transform your life. Most of you can experience remarkable improvement over a short period of time, irrespective of your age or medical condition.

2. Just Do It!

Although most people wait until they are sick before they seek medical attention, I now see more and more "healthy" patients who do not have any specific diagnosable disease. My typical "healthy" patient is in his or her forties or fifties and is seeking my help not to treat a specific problem but to heal a variety of subtle ailments before they become acute. Typically, these patients sense that they are entering a stage of decline and are somewhat alarmed about what is happening to their bodies. They are concerned because they have put on weight and are losing muscle tone. They step out of the shower one morning, catch a glimpse of themselves in the mirror, and realize that their body is not as well toned or strong as it used to be. Most are surprised by how tired and drained they feel at the end of the day. They frequently have other concerns as well. Men and women alike tell me (sometimes reluctantly) that they are uninterested in sex or feel too tired to even think about it. In fact, quite a number of men—many more than you would guess—say they have experienced bouts of impotence. Yet the most frequent complaint that I hear is this: "Dr. Whitaker, I just don't understand it. I'm not doing anything differently, but I just can't seem to do what I used to do."

What these patients don't realize is that they are diagnosing their problem with remarkable clarity and accuracy. The problem is that even though *they* are not doing anything differently, *their bodies* are doing many things differently. They look and feel worn out because their bodies are running differently and in some cases running down. They, in turn, are not doing anything different to compensate for it. I explain that they have begun to *age,* that what is going on outside their bodies is very much a reflection of what is going on inside. The problem is more than "skin deep." I also hasten to add that all is not lost, that their situation is not hopeless, and that the age-related changes they are sensing are not irreversible. I then explain that in order to reverse what is happening, they must first understand why it is happening.

HOW THE YEARS CREEP UP ON US

At about the time we reach age forty, our bodies begin to undergo profound changes that affect every aspect of our lives, including how we look, how we feel, how we think, and, in

18

sum, *how we age.* This "midlife slump" begins with a decline in the body's energy-producing system. For most people one of the first signs of middle age is excessive fatigue. Just think about how many times you have heard someone, including yourself, say, "I feel as if I'm running out of steam." This actually is a very apt description of what is happening inside our cells as we age and a very apt description of the aging process itself.

Every human activity—even breathing and thinking—requires energy. To satisfy this demand, our bodies function as energy-producing factories. Energy production is a very complicated process that works essentially like this: It begins with the food we eat, which is digested or broken down into smaller components in the gastrointestinal tract. After the food is digested, it must be metabolized, or broken down even further into a form that can be utilized by the cells of the body for energy—in other words, into fuel. This fuel is converted into energy by tiny structures called mitochondria, which are the "power plants" inside our cells. As we age, the mitochondria begin to run down and lose their ability to produce energy as well or as efficiently.

This energy shortage affects every cell and system in our body. The heart, the brain, and the kidneys slow down. Cells lose their ability to repair themselves and die. Our immune system functions less efficiently. Our endocrine system stops producing hormones at youthful levels. Our skin dries out. And perhaps the most visible consequence of this midlife energy shortage is that our metabolism slows down, making it more difficult to burn calories. As a result we store fat, put on weight, and lose muscle tone.

Another, more complex cause of this energy drain is the decline in our antioxidant defense network that occurs at midlife. Although oxygen is essential for life, it is ironic that constant exposure to oxygen accelerates aging. Oxygen triggers the formation of dangerously unstable molecular fragments known as "free radicals." Free radicals bind easily with other molecules, and when they do, they can damage healthy tissue. Free radicals can also attack the DNA or genetic material within the nucleus of the cell, causing it to mutate and become cancerous. Fortunately, our bodies have an elaborate built-in defense system that works to repel these attacks. For instance, every cell produces substances called antioxidants that neutralize free radicals before they can run amuck. Food also contains other important antioxidants such as beta-carotene, vitamins C and E, and selenium that we do not produce within our bodies.

When we are young, we have sufficient antioxidant stores to keep free radicals in check. As we age, however, our levels of naturally produced antioxidants decline, and at middle age we experience a particularly steep drop in the body's primary antioxidant, glutathione. From that point on we live in a chronic state of antioxidant deficit, which continues as we age.

The cumulative effects of the energy drain and the loss of our antioxidant advantage are obvious and devastating. They are the proximate cause of almost every illness commonly associated with aging, including obesity and adult onset diabetes, heart disease, Alzheimer's disease, and arthritis. They even cause wrinkles.

When we reach this point in our lives, we have a choice to make. We can simply accept these changes philosophically as the inevitable consequences of aging and not respond to our body's changing needs. Or we can intervene and take steps to help our bodies meet and overcome these new challenges, which in turn will slow the rate at which we age and reverse much of the damage that aging already has inflicted.

Think of two new cars. They both roll off the assembly line at precisely the same time. One car is delivered to an owner who is a careless driver, who rarely takes the car in for scheduled oil changes and tune-ups, who fills the tank with low-octane fuel, and who leaves the car outside no matter what the weather. Ten years and one hundred thousand miles later—perhaps even sooner—the car is ready for the junk heap.

The second car, however, is purchased by a careful driver who is conscientious about maintenance. He fills the car with premium gasoline, takes it in for scheduled maintenance, and wouldn't dream of leaving it outside in bad weather. Moreover, as the car gets older, he takes it in for service at shorter intervals, maybe every three thousand instead of every five thousand miles. Ten years and one hundred thousand miles later, this car still looks and runs like a dream.

The human body is similar to a car in that it, too, is a complex piece of machinery that requires the right maintenance at the right times. Maintenance can make a huge difference in how our minds and our bodies, like our automobiles, last. If we practice maximum maintenance, we can actually slow the pace at which we age.

Of course, I do not discount other factors, such as genetics, that also play a role in how we age. There will always be folks who seem to live forever not because of how they take care of themselves but in spite of it. You've probably heard of the 120-year-old woman in France who didn't give up smoking until she was 100, or the great-great-grandfather who consumed large amounts of bacon and eggs every morning, drank heavily, at age 80 fathered a child, and lived to be 105. Certainly, some people do age better than others because they are genetically programmed for exceptional good health and longevity. Most of us, however, are not that fortunate. We are programmed to age "normally," meaning that by middle age we will begin to show signs of wear and tear, and begin to *feel* as well as show our age. What's worse is that through neglect and inaction, most of us actually accelerate the aging process.

To employ my automobile analogy again, consider how a skillful mechanic can perform wonders on a used car. In relatively short order an old clunker can be refitted with new parts, molded into shape, and recharged. With proper servicing, the car can look and drive almost like new, and if cared for, it can stay in peak condition for a long time. I want you to think of my Age Loss Program as the ultimate tune-up for your body and your mind. Over the course of the next ten weeks you will be the mechanic who performs wonders on yourself. You will mold your body into shape, tune up your internal environment, and erase a decade's worth of damage. In ten weeks you will feel—and be—recharged, revved up, and ready for life. You will have added a good ten years—a very good ten years—to your life. This is what *Shed Ten Years in Ten Weeks* is all about.

I want to stress that my Age Loss Program is not only highly effective but also highly enjoyable. I promise you that the next ten weeks of your life will be a pleasure, not a struggle. You will not feel deprived or unhappy; you will not feel that you could or should be doing better things with your time.

One of the guiding principles of my practice is that you cannot make people miserable in the name of good health. You cannot expect people to starve themselves, eat bad-tasting food, exercise to exhaustion, or turn their lives upside down. If you do, they will just throw in the towel and retreat to their old habits. That will not happen with the Age Loss Program. I have patients who have stayed on my program for close to two decades because it has helped them reclaim their health and they actually enjoy it.

Shed Ten Years in Ten Weeks consists of ten steps, each one designed to strengthen the body and mind in very specific ways. You do not have to follow every step to get results. Each step is powerful in its own right, and you will reap benefits from following any one of them. Yet I believe they work best synergistically. If you want to get the full ten-year advantage, I urge you to complete the entire ten-step program. Here is a quick breakdown of what each step will do for you.

STEP 1: ALL SYSTEMS GO!

This *easy* over-the-counter Rx will allow you to shed ten years and rev up your body! You will begin the Age Loss Program with a jump start in the form of new high-tech supplements that will reenergize your body and tune up your metabolism. These over-the-counter supplements will help you burn fat, build muscle, and renew your antioxidant defense system quickly, safely, and effectively.

STEP 2: LOSE A DECADE'S WORTH OF FAT

When we reach middle age, we gain on average about ten pounds of fat a decade. By combining the correct foods with the right supplements, the Age Loss Program's food plan can restore metabolic function to more youthful levels, enabling our bodies to burn fat before it is stored as extra pounds. This diet will enable you to lose ten years of fat in ten weeks . . . and keep it off.

STEP 3: SHED TEN YEARS' WORTH OF FINE LINES AND WRINKLES—RENEW TIRED, WORN-OUT SKIN

This comprehensive skin care regimen will show you how supplements, food, lifestyle changes, and state-of-the-art skin creams can renew your skin from the inside out and the outside in. At the end of ten weeks you will see radiant, resilient skin that glows with health and vitality.

STEP 4: REGAIN TEN YEARS OF MUSCLE

From age forty on, the typical adult loses lean body mass or muscle with every passing decade. Step 4 is a quick, simple, and effective way to turn a flabby body into a strong, sleek body in just ten weeks, without undue exertion or stress on your body. Designed by an exercise physiologist for the Whitaker Wellness Institute, the Age Loss Program's exercise routines use techniques employed by world-class athletes to achieve maximum results in minimum time, but they are simplified and refined for us to use at home.

STEP 5: BOOST YOUR BRAIN POWER

Age-related changes in your brain are causing a subtle but very real decline in mental function. From age forty on, we experience dramatic changes in short-term memory, we have greater difficulty concentrating for long periods of time, and we have a harder time learning new things. Step 5 provides you with simple but highly effective ways to sharpen your mental edge and maximize brain function.

STEP 6: REVITALIZE YOUR SEX LIFE

Step 6 explains how to prevent and reverse the most common sexual problems for men and women. Thanks to new treatments (some of the best are sold over the counter) and technological breakthroughs, almost everyone can enjoy an active and sometimes even better sex life well into their 60s and 70s and even beyond.

STEP 7: REJUVENATE WHILE YOU SLEEP

Every good night's sleep is like a mini vacation. Sleep recharges and reinvigorates every important system within the body, from your ability to cope with stress to your ability to ward off infection. A good night's sleep can be one of nature's most rejuvenating experiences. Step 7 explains how you can maximize the power of sleep.

STEP 8: RECHARGE THE SPIRIT

The Age Loss Program is not just about a strong body and a sharp mind; it is about renewal of the spirit and recapturing the kind of joie de vivre that makes life worth living. Stress and the grind of daily living can sap us of our joy of life and make us forget what life is all about. Step 8 shows you how to feed the soul and make your spirits soar.

STEP 9: REINVIGORATE YOUR IMMUNE SYSTEM

One of the first signs of aging is difficulty in shaking off a common cold or flu virus. Our vulnerability to illness is caused by age-related changes in our immune system, which grows weaker with each passing year. Step 9 of the Age Loss

Program introduces some novel techniques to strengthen the body's "weak link," to promote health and longevity.

STEP 10: REGAIN A DECADE'S WORTH OF HEALTH BY CORRECTING THE GLITCHES

With each passing decade we experience changes in vital body systems, which can cause disease. Step 10 of the Age Loss Program addresses the needs of people with special health concerns and provides an Rx for treating and reversing such common health problems as osteoarthritis, diabetes, high blood pressure, heart disease, and loss of vision.

READY ... SET ... GO!

Before you begin the Age Loss Program, I want to share with you some final thoughts.

We are not the first generation that has attempted to slow the aging process, but we are certainly the first generation that has *succeeded*.

As many of you know, hundreds of years ago Ponce de León went on a costly and dangerous journey through the swamps of Florida in search of the legendary fountain of youth. Until very recently the concept of reversing aging has been shrouded in myth and superstition. But keep in mind that years ago the concept of curing disease seemed to be a myth as well. There was a time when it was believed that disease was caused by supernatural forces. Intervention was regarded as pointless and foolish—tempting the gods.

Today we have as rational an understanding of aging as we have of disease. We are learning how to slow and even reverse the aging process. There is a body of solid, compelling scientific research which shows unequivocally that life can be not only extended well beyond what we ever thought possible but also that our health and destiny are very much in our own hands.

And now you are ready to begin the best ten weeks of your life.

Step 1

ALL SYSTEMS GO!

Jump-start the rejuvenation process
Recharge your batteries
Regain a decade's worth of energy and endurance

When I turned fifty, I noticed some real changes in how I felt and I how I looked. I used to be on the go all the time, but then I fatigued more easily. I simply couldn't keep up with my usual schedule. What I found even more distressing was that I was beginning to feel a few aches and pains from arthritis. My skin was drier and was looking "old." I was very worried that it was going to be downhill from here. Within a month after I started on Dr. Whitaker's supplement regimen, I noticed a real increase in energy. I felt terrific; the aches and pains had vanished. What surprised me was the fact that I looked so much better: My skin glowed with good health. . . . The best part is, I keep getting better and better.

ELLEN, 52, SAN FRANCISCO, CALIFORNIA

ELLEN'S STORY IS TYPICAL of those that I hear from my patients who have been following my comprehensive high-tech supplement plan specifically designed to arrest the energy drain that saps our bodies of strength and vitality and makes us age before our time. Restoring energy is the key to reclaiming our health and vitality. That is why it is Step 1 of my Age Loss Program.

Each step of my Age Loss Program is important, but I consider my high-tech supplements the cornerstone. Supplements are essential for slowing down the forces that accelerate aging, and that is what *Shed Ten Years in Ten Weeks* is all about. Follow my supplement regimen for the full ten weeks of the Age Loss Program, and you will be delighted with the results.

Fortunately, taking supplements is something we all can do no matter how busy. I will show you how to make it as much a part of your daily routine as brushing your teeth.

With all the supplements that are on the market today, I understand that figuring out which ones to use and in what doses to use them can be thoroughly confusing. On page 48 I provide you with a shopping list of the supplements that you will need, along with instructions on how to use them.

I can attest to the incredible power of supplements from my own personal experience. I credit the Age Loss Program's method of using supplements with giving me the strength I need, at age fifty-three, to see a constant stream of patients, handle medical emergencies, write books and a monthly newsletter, lecture all over the world, and take an active part in the lives of my wonderful children.

The Age Loss Program's supplement plan also helped me achieve what appeared to be an impossible dream for a man my age: cycling across the United States. At the age of fifty-one I joined a group of cyclists and pedaled coast to coast, from Bellingham, Washington, to Washington, D.C. The ride was ten weeks long and covered well over four thousand miles. What is remarkable about this is that cycling was never my usual form of exercise. I had only four months to train, and that was not enough time for the rigorous trip ahead. I knew that I needed an extra boost to get me up to speed. In addition to the supplements I took daily, I added two energy-boosting supplements: potassium magnesium aspartate, which improves stamina, and creatine monohydrate, which builds muscle.

On our trip we rode all day long and averaged sixty to eighty miles a day, but sometimes we rode over one hundred miles! The first week we crossed the Cascade Mountains, climbing steep grades that were difficult even for cars. The experience would have been challenging even for the most avid cyclist, let alone a novice like me. At first I was one of the slowest riders in the group, managing only ten miles per hour. After cycling for four or five hours, I was exhausted and ready to call it a day. I am proud to say, however, that by mid-trip I was one of the strongest riders, leading the pack at a brisk seventeen to eighteen miles per hour. I was on the road every morning before 8:00 A.M. and still going strong when evening rolled around. I was amazed at what I was able to accomplish in just a few weeks!

I credit this feat in part to the supplements I took. Of course, physical conditioning and the right food also helped increase my strength and stamina, but these unique supplements gave me the edge I needed.

Although you may not be doing anything nearly as physically demanding as cycling cross-country, over the next ten weeks, you will be working with your body in new ways. Your body will be working hard to restore itself, and it will need the fuel to accomplish this important task. That is why my program incorporates the same energy-boosting supplements that I used on my ten-week bicycle trip.

THE RDAs ALONE ARE NOT ENOUGH

Most of you have probably heard of the government RDAs, or Recommended Daily Allowances for vitamins and minerals set by the National Academy of Sciences. Along with a substantial and growing number of scientists and physicians, I consider the RDAs ridiculously low.

In reality, the RDAs have little to do with health and everything to do with illness. The RDAs represent the government's determination of the bare *minimum* amount of certain vitamins and minerals we need to consume each day in order to prevent deficiency diseases such as scurvy (caused by a shortage of vitamin C) or beriberi (caused by a shortage of thiamine, a B vitamin). The truth is, most of us don't even think about these diseases anymore because they are quite rare in the Western world. When most of us take our vitamins, we think about maintaining our health. The problem with the RDAs is that they do not tell us what we need in order to enjoy *optimum* health and vitality. Nor do the RDAs account for the fact that we all are different and have differing nutritional needs.

Furthermore, the RDAs are outmoded. They were compiled more than half a century ago when scientists knew very little about how our cells worked and how micronutrients and cells interact. Today we know that vitamins, minerals, phytochemicals (disease-fighting compounds found in plants), enzymes, and other essential substances found in food do more than protect us from diseases such as scurvy. They play a key role in *preventing* many diseases, including cancer, heart disease, and even depression.

Study after study has clearly documented that when blood levels of vitamins, minerals, and other important micronutrients drop below optimal levels, our bodies cannot function properly. This doesn't mean that each time we forget to take our supplements we will immediately display symptoms of a deficiency or disease. But consistent failure to take them will eventually catch up with us. When it does, our bodies will weaken, we will become more susceptible to disease, and we will *age faster.*

The Age Loss Program's method of using supplements is based on what I call the *optimal daily allowance,* or "ODA," for each vitamin and mineral. My goal is to achieve and maintain optimum good health and vitality, not simply prevent a deficiency disease. As you may notice, whole categories of supplements not even listed in the RDAs are utilized, including essential fatty acids (omega-3 oils) and potent herbs such as ginkgo biloba. If you follow my Age Loss ODAs, you can be assured that you are getting the right supplements in amounts that will satisfy most of your needs and fortify your body against the slowdown in key systems that promotes disease and accelerates aging. The supplements will have an immediate and positive impact on your health and your life. The sooner you begin the Age Loss Program's supplement plan, the sooner you will begin to reap the rewards. You will feel stronger, more vigorous, and even happier.

Since I prescribe dosages that are much higher than the RDAs, I am frequently asked whether one can "overdose" on supplements. The answer is NO! The dosages that I prescribe are safe and effective, and have been used by thousands of patients. You will not have any problems if you stick to my recommended doses.

My Age Loss ODAs can be taken by everyone. The plan is designed for men and women who, though experiencing the symptoms we associate with aging—such as weight gain, fatigue, loss of muscle tone and flexibility, mild memory loss or poor concentration, joint stiffness, dry skin, and wrinkles —are not acutely ill. Throughout the book I also recommend some additional supplements for men and women to meet special needs.

If you have specific health problems, however, such as high blood pressure, high cholesterol, heart disease, or diabetes, you should refer to Step 10 to find out if additional supplements are in order. And, of course, those of you who have these problems should be under a doctor's supervision.

• • •

Before you start the plan, I want to tell you about each supplement you will be taking. You are probably familiar with many of the supplements that comprise my program but not all of them, especially the new state-of-the-art supplements that I use routinely but that are not yet well known to the public. Therefore, I feel it is important for you to understand the benefits of each supplement. For your convenience I have also included a chart on page 49 listing each supplement along with my ODA.

Essential Fatty Acids

Essential fatty acids are "good fats" that are necessary for many important body functions, and they protect against both heart disease and cancer. Unfortunately, our diet is lopsided: It is high in bad fat that can cause disease, and low in the essential fats that can prevent disease and keep us young. Omega-3 fatty acids derived from fish oil are an excellent source of essential fatty acids. (Greater detail about the role of essential fatty acids is given in Step 2.) Because we are so deficient in essential fatty acids, I recommend that you take 1,000 milligrams of omega-3 fatty acids daily. Omega-3 fatty acids contain two good essential fatty acids: eicosapantaenoic acid (EPA) and decosahexaenoic acid (DHA). Be sure the supplement contains 360 milligrams of EPA and 240 milligrams DHA.

Omega-3 fatty acids are natural blood thinners. If you are taking any medication to thin your blood, do not take omega-3 fatty acids without consulting your physician.

The Antioxidants: Maintaining the Youthful Balance

My Age Loss Program's supplement plan includes generous doses of antioxidants, such as vitamin A, beta-carotene, and the mineral selenium (all of which should be in your multivitamin in sufficient quantities), and vitamins C, E, lipoic acid, and the herb ginkgo biloba (which you will probably have to obtain separately). Antioxidants can prevent free radicals from causing cellular damage. Some antioxidants, known as free radical scavengers, patrol the body, blocking the formation of free radicals. Other antioxidants disarm the already formed free radicals before they can bind with other molecules. Let me give a brief description of some of the most important antioxidants in the Age Loss ODAs.

Vitamin A Found in eggs and liver, vitamin A is essential for healthy skin and eyes. Numerous studies have shown that vitamin A is effective against many different types of cancer, particularly oral cancers. The Age Loss ODA for vitamin A is 5,000 IU. (Vitamin A will be in your high-potency multivitamin.)

Beta-carotene Found in leafy green and yellow fruits and vegetables, beta-carotene is converted into vitamin A as the body needs it. Beta-carotene is a potent antioxidant that is well known for its ability to protect against both cancer and heart disease. I recommend 15,000 IU of beta-carotene daily. (Beta-carotene will be in your high-potency multivitamin.)

Vitamin C Essential for the formation of collagen, vitamin C is necessary for the production of new cells and tissue. In 1970, Dr. Linus Pauling's book, *Vitamin C and the Common Cold*, rocked the medical establishment by suggesting that high doses of vitamin C (well beyond the RDA of 60 milligrams) could shorten the length and severity of a cold. We now know that vitamin C relieves the symptoms of a cold by reducing the histamine level in your bloodstream; histamines are what cause the runny nose and watery eyes typical of colds. Over the past two decades we have learned some truly remarkable things about vitamin C that go well beyond its role as a treatment for colds. Studies have shown that vitamin C can protect against several types of common cancers and heart disease. The Age Loss ODA is 2,500 milligrams (You will probably have to supplement your multivitamin with vitamin C.)

Vitamin E Researchers are discovering new and exciting uses for vitamin E almost daily. Recently, two important studies showed that high doses of vitamin E (well beyond the RDA of 10 milligrams) can strengthen immune function in older people and slow the progression of Alzheimer's disease more effectively than drugs. Vitamin E can also reduce the risk of heart disease and is even used as a treatment for hot flashes during menopause. The Age Loss ODA is 800 milligrams. You will probably have to supplement your multivitamin with vitamin E. (Vitamin E is a natural blood thinner. If you are taking medication to thin your blood, do not take vitamin E supplements without consulting your physician.)

Selenium This mineral protects against stroke and has recently been shown to reduce dramatically the incidence of serious cancers in people who took at least 200 micrograms daily, which is more than three times the RDA. You will probably have to supplement your multivitamin with selenium. (The Age Loss ODA for selenium is 200 micrograms, and you will find it in most good high-potency multivitamins.)

Ginkgo biloba Derived from the ginkgo tree, this herb can improve circulation throughout the body and is well known for its ability to enhance memory. (You will learn more about ginkgo biloba in Steps 5 and 6.) There is no RDA for ginkgo biloba. The Age Loss ODA is 120 milligrams, so you will probably have to supplement your multivitamin with ginkgo biloba.

In addition to antioxidants we get through food and supplements, our bodies also produce natural antioxidants such as glutathione, superoxide dismutase, and lipoic acid. (More information about lipoic acid, a unique "energizing antioxidant," will be found on page 39.) Our naturally produced antioxidants decline with age and with disease.

Restoring and maintaining the proper antioxidant balance in your body is key to the rejuvenation process, and age loss will not happen without it.

Antioxidants come in all different forms, and supplements cannot do the job alone. In Step 2 I show you simple ways to increase your antioxidant intake through food. In Step 3 I also recommend potent antioxidant creams that help restore the antioxidant balance in the skin. But for now, let's concentrate on antioxidant supplements.

The antioxidants we consume through supplements and food also work in synergy with the antioxidants that our bodies produce naturally. Both vitamin C and lipoic acid supplements can increase levels of glutathione, the body's natural defense mechanism against free radicals. This is of great importance since glutathione levels fall as we age, and glutathione supplements are difficult to absorb. Increasing our intake of vitamin C and lipoic acid supplements, which are easily absorbed by the body, can give us the glutathione boost we need to tip the odds in our favor in the war against free radicals.

Although each antioxidant plays a unique role, they are meant to work together in a unified network. Each antioxidant enhances the action of the other, and when combined, they form a juggernaut against free radicals.

AGE SAVER: An Investment of a Few Seconds a Day (the Time It Takes to Swallow a Pill) Can Add Years to Your Life

Researchers at the University of California examined the vitamin C intakes and death rates of more than eleven thousand men and women. They found that those who took vitamin C supplements well above the RDA lived an average of six years longer!

THE ENERGIZERS: LIPOIC ACID, CHROMIUM PICOLINATE, COENZYME Q-10, AND POTASSIUM-MAGNESIUM ASPARTATE

One common symptom of aging is a loss of energy and a feeling of fatigue. Therefore, I have included four supplements that I call The Energizers to recharge your battery.

The Energizers are a select group of natural substances that enhance the bioenergetic system and help us use energy more efficiently. The midlife energy slump that is part of the aging process is very much a result of the wearing down of the body's energy system. The net effect is that as we age, our bodies are being called upon to do the same amount of work with less and less energy. The supplements I call The Energizers achieve their effect by restoring the body's energy system and enhancing the body's ability to either produce or utilize energy.

The Energizers not only restore flagging pep and endurance but also play a larger role. The Energizers strengthen every system in your body, including your immune system, your cardiovascular system, and your nervous system. The Energizers also work together to rev up metabolism. As a

38

result, you will lose fat, gain lean body mass, and achieve a trimmer, sleeker body. Operating in tandem with my Age Loss cuisine and exercise routine, The Energizers will have a dramatic impact on how you look and feel.

Lipoic Acid: The "Hottest" Energizing Antioxidant

Lipoic acid, which has only just begun to appear on the shelves of health food stores, is also instrumental in maintaining the energy system of the body. Lipoic acid is naturally produced in the body, but as we age, we stop producing it in sufficient quantities. This is why I believe we need to take lipoic acid supplements.

I am very excited about the possibilities of lipoic acid and predict that this extraordinary supplement will soon get all the attention it deserves. Dr. Lester Packer, a world-renowned scientist who heads the Membrane Bioenergetics Group at the University of California at Berkeley, discovered that lipoic acid differs from other antioxidants in several important ways. First, unlike other antioxidants that have a specific job in the body, lipoic acid is so versatile that it can serve as a "free agent" and pinch-hit for the other antioxidants when they are in short supply. In other words, if you are low in vitamin E or C, lipoic acid will temporarily take over the vitamins' jobs. Second, and perhaps most important, lipoic acid greatly enhances the potency of vitamins C and E. Combined with lipoic acid, these two antioxidants are more powerful and their beneficial effects more long-lasting than when they stand alone.

Despite its benefits, lipoic acid is only now getting some of the recognition it deserves. More than two decades ago Dr. Burton Berkson, then a medical resident, reported that lipoic acid could cure a fatal liver disease caused by the ingestion of highly poisonous aminita mushrooms. Sixty to 90 percent of people who eat this toxic mushroom die. But scientists found that lipoic acid cured these patients. Despite its great promise, a therapeutic tool for liver problems, most scientists stopped studying it. Why? Good question. I can only assume that it is because lipoic is a natural substance and therefore, since it cannot be patented, no pharmaceutical company has the economic incentive to champion its cause.

Thankfully for us, some steadfast scientists such as Dr. Packer have continued their work on lipoic acid, and their discoveries are making it impossible for the medical establishment to ignore lipoic acid any longer. In fact, scientists now know that lipoic acid raises metabolism. Athletes, body builders, and others who need extra energy to maintain their strength and stamina are already taking lipoic acid supplements. It increases energy production in muscle cells and at the same time its antioxidant action reduces the soreness and stiffness that frequently accompany a rigorous workout.

And that's not all lipoic acid does. One of the most important functions of lipoic acid is to normalize blood sugar levels. High blood sugar is a common problem for many middle-aged and older men and women because they develop insulin resistance (also known as Type II diabetes). This condition affects some 16 million Americans. Insulin is the hormone that helps break down sugar or glucose so that it can be utilized by the cells of the body. If you are resistant to insulin, you will have higher than normal levels of blood sugar or glucose, which is problematic for several reasons.

First, it prevents nutrients from getting into cells, depriving them of the raw material needed to make energy. Second, glucose is a magnet for free radicals, which can destroy healthy tissue throughout the body. Over time, high blood sugar levels can result in serious health problems such as atherosclerosis (hardening of the arteries), nerve damage, and blindness. In fact, lipoic acid has been used quite successfully in Europe for several decades to prevent complications from insulin resistance and other forms of diabetes, but it has been virtually ignored in the United States. But it won't be for much longer, I predict. (The Age Loss ODA for lipoic acid is 50 milligrams daily.)

Chromium Picolinate: The Body's Top Anti-Sugar Cop

Another exceptional supplement that is growing in popularity is chromium picolinate. The effect of chromium picolinate is truly astounding, and I can assure you that if it were a patented drug rather than an inexpensive over-the-counter supplement, we would hear a great deal more about it.

Chromium picolinate burns fat, increases muscle mass, and, like lipoic acid, is an excellent treatment for insulin resistance. Chromium picolinate also lowers blood cholesterol levels while raising the level of "good" cholesterol, or HDL. There is even evidence that this remarkable mineral has control over the hypothalamus, the "satiety center" of the brain which signals to us that we have had enough to eat and that it is time to stop eating. Unfortunately, most Americans are seriously chromium deficient, and I believe that this is one of the reasons that insulin resistance and obesity are so common here.

Chromium is considered a trace mineral because it is used in minute quantities by the body. Chromium is better absorbed when combined with the metal picolinate than when taken alone. Since most of our food supply is heavily processed and refined, with the result that many trace minerals such as chromium are stripped away, it is nearly impossible to get adequate chromium from food alone. To make matters worse, studies have shown that a high sugar diet— the kind that most Americans eat—saps the body of chromium. In fact, 90 percent of all Americans do not even consume the 50 micrograms per day of chromium that the National Academy of Sciences recommends.

For many years I have used chromium with great success to treat patients suffering from Type II or insulin resistance diabetes. Chromium makes the cells more insulin friendly, thereby helping to keep blood sugar levels under control.

Chromium is also especially useful for people who need to lose fat but not muscle. This is demonstrated by an important study undertaken at the Health and Medical Research Foundation of San Antonio, Texas. One group of overweight volunteers took 200 to 400 micrograms of chromium daily and made no other changes in their lifestyle. Another group took a placebo. After seventy-one days, the chromium group had lost an average of 4.2 pounds of body fat; those in the control group lost a scant four-tenths of a pound. The chromium group also gained 1.4 pounds of lean muscle, and the control group gained none. Needless to say, chromium produces even better results when combined with the Age Loss Program's food plan and workout routines. (The Age Loss ODA for chromium picolinate is 200 micrograms daily.)

Coenzyme Q10:
The Cellular Spark Plug That Revs Up the Cells

Co-Q10 is essential to the body's energy extraction mechanism. Much like spark plugs are needed to jump-start an engine, Co-Q10 provides the spark without which the body cannot run.

Blood levels of Co-Q10 decline as we age, and the effects of this decline are profound. Dr. Karl Folkers, the renowned scientist who first synthesized Co-Q10, has hypothesized that a widespread deficiency of Co-Q10 may be responsible for the epidemic of congestive heart failure in the United States. This makes perfect sense since heart failure, which is now a leading cause of death in the United States, results from the inability of the heart to generate the energy and strength necessary to maintain adequate circulation.

Many studies, including several published in the distinguished *American Journal of Cardiology,* confirm that Co-Q10 is an excellent treatment for heart disease. One of these studies showed that Co-Q10 can increase stamina and reduce angina (chest pain) in heart patients undergoing an exercise treadmill test. What is particularly important about this finding is that exercise is one of the most effective treatments for heart disease, yet many heart patients are reluctant to exercise because when they do, they experience chest pain.

In another study, Dr. Peter Langsjoen, a Texas cardiologist compared the progress of heart patients who were taking only standard cardiac drugs to patients who were also taking Co-Q10. *Remarkably, the patients taking the Co-Q10 lived an average of more than three years longer.* In other words, simply by taking this inexpensive supplement, heart patients were adding years to their lives. The role of Co-Q10 in promoting heart health is no longer surprising to me and the researchers who have studied it. What I do find surprising is how few doctors bother to prescribe it.

High doses of Co-Q10 are being used to treat advanced cancer, including breast cancer, with much success. This doesn't surprise me, either. When the body has adequate energy, every organ and system can perform well, and the body is generally more able to fight disease and heal itself.

However, don't get the idea that Co-Q10 is just for people who are sick or who are suffering from heart disease. We all need it in sufficient levels. If we are Co-Q10 deficient, we will not have the strength and stamina to live a full and active life. So why haven't you heard about Co-Q10 from your doctor, and why isn't it included in the RDAs?

Once again we need to talk bottom line. When Dr. Folkers was a research scientist at Merck, Sharpe and Dohme, the pharmaceutical giant, he synthesized Co-Q10. Dr. Folkers recognized the potential of Co-Q10 as a life saver. However, because Co-Q10 is a natural substance that cannot be patented, the company had no economic incentive to pursue the research further. Instead, the company sold the technology for synthesizing Co-Q10 to Japan. As a result, Dr. Folkers left Merck in the late 1960s to research Co-Q10 full-time. America's loss was Japan's gain. Today there are 6 million Japanese taking this inexpensive but highly effective supplement, while few here in the United States have even heard about it.

Unfortunately for Americans, this is a pattern that is repeated over and over again. European and Asian countries are light-years ahead of us in terms of the willingness of their medical establishments to use natural, inexpensive remedies that work. (I recommend 60 milligrams of Co-Q10 daily.)

Potassium-Magnesium Aspartate: The Dynamic Trio for Strength and Stamina

Potassium and magnesium are two well-known minerals that perform many different jobs in the body. When combined with the amino acid aspartate, they become a true energizing compound that stimulates increased production of ATP, the body's fuel. As far back as the 1960s, researchers discovered that potassium-magnesium aspartate can dramatically increase physical endurance. One study published in a leading Scandinavian medical journal, for example, tested the effects of potassium-magnesium aspartate on six physically fit men. For four consecutive days the men exercised on a stationary bicycle until exhausted. On the first two days and the last day, they took placebo tablets, but on the third day they were given potassium-magnesium aspartate. On the day that the men took placebos, they were able to exercise an average of

85.3 minutes. Yet remarkably, on the day they took potassium-magnesium aspartate, they were able to exercise for 128 minutes, a 50 percent increase! Given the astounding success rate, word about potassium-magnesium aspartate spread quickly among serious athletes. As noted earlier, I, too, started using potassium-magnesium aspartate when I was training for my cross-country bicycle trip to help build up my endurance, and within days I experienced a real difference in stamina.

If you still aren't convinced, here is another success story. A friend of mine who rides his bicycle eight miles each morning complained to me that he found the last two miles particularly difficult and often experienced pain in his upper and lower legs. I recommended that he try potassium-magnesium aspartate. He later wrote me a letter and reported, "The result was amazing and immediate. I was able to increase my average speed (15 mph) over the same course to 18 mph with none of the muscle fatigue that I had experienced before. I am able to ride the first 2.68 miles of the course 5 mph faster than previously."

Even if you are not a serious athlete, I recommend that you take potassium-magnesium aspartate daily for two reasons: First, it will give you an energy boost and increase your stamina so that you will have the endurance you need to work out effectively. Second, it will help you shed fat faster and more efficiently. As you've undoubtedly heard for years, one of the best ways to maintain your weight is to burn calories through exercise, and potassium-magnesium aspartate will help you exercise for a longer period of time without suffering from excess fatigue. To get the maximum benefit of potassium-magnesium aspartate, you should do at least some regular moderate exercise at least three times a week. Besides, I guarantee that after taking this supplement, you will have so much energy that you will actually want to exercise! (The recommended dose is 1,000 milligrams daily.)

THE MUSCLE BUILDER: CREATINE MONOHYDRATE

At around forty years old, we begin to lose muscle and gain fat, resulting in a loss of body tone and definition. In other words, we become flabby.

Exercise will help restore muscle, but if you want to recover the muscle that you have lost over the past decade, you need to do more. That is why I recommend that you use this special muscle-building supplement, creatine monohydrate, for the first four weeks of the Age Loss Program. Creatine can have such a remarkable effect on the body's ability to repair and regenerate muscle that I'd like to tell you more about this terrific supplement.

Creatine is already popular among body builders and athletes who want to enhance their muscle strength but who are unwilling to subject themselves to anabolic steroids, which are illegal (unless medically prescribed) and can have terrible and potentially fatal side effects. Creatine does not. It will help you achieve a stronger, sleeker, and healthier body, safely and effectively, without dangerous side effects.

Creatine is a protein that occurs naturally in our bodies. About 95 percent of the body's creatine is found in skeletal muscles. Heavy concentrations of creatine are found in the male testes where sperm is stored, and the rest is distributed throughout the body.

Creatine is essential for the production of ATP, the fuel that runs the body and jump-starts the cells. Creatine monohydrate is the form of creatine used in supplements because it is the most stable and is best absorbed by the body. Creatine monohydrate supplements provide an energy boost that enables you to work out harder and for a longer period of time. Several studies have shown that by combining exercise with creatine monohydrate supplements, you will gain more muscle and lose more fat than by exercise alone. It also builds muscle even if you don't exercise, but when combined with exercise, the effects are far more dramatic.

Creatine is also found in food, especially meat and fish, and on average we consume about 1 gram of creatine daily from our diet. Vegetarians and people who do not eat a lot of meat generally have low levels of creatine and may need to obtain it by supplement even at a young age.

My recommended dose for creatine monohydrate is found on page 50, but keep in mind that on the days you exercise it is best to take creatine monohydrate immediately after your workout since it will help muscles repair more quickly.

GO GREEN WITH GREEN DRINKS

Green Drinks are a new class of nutritional supplements derived from the juices of young green plants and are sold by mail order and in health food stores. Green drinks consist of a base of wheat or barley grass juice. Young greens are packed with phytochemicals, and are a rich source of vitamins, minerals, and a number of protective antioxidants and enzymes. Since most of us do not get enough greens in our diet, I strongly recommend that you drink one green drink daily to fill this nutritional gap.

Green drinks are sold as powders, which can be mixed in water or juice. The ODA for green drinks is three teaspoons of powdered greens mixed in eight ounces of water or juice, taken on an empty stomach.

There are a number of excellent brands of green drinks, including Fiber Greens + from Healthy Directions, Inc. (my own mail order brand) or these products can be obtained through health food stores; Greens + from Orange Peel Enterprises; Green Magna from Green Foods and Kyo-Green from Wakunaga of America.

YOUR DAILY SUPPLEMENT PLAN FOR WEEKS ONE TO TEN

Now you are familiar with the supplements that you will be taking for the next ten weeks and the daily dosage for each one. To make it simple for you, I have put together a list of supplements for you to buy. All the supplements I recommend can be purchased at health food stores, pharmacies, and by mail order. Use the shopping list below to make sure you are buying the right supplements. They are available in pills, capsules, powdered drinks, and even in flavored chewable wafer form. Unless I specify otherwise, choose the form that you find easiest to take.

In the interest of full disclosure I do have to note that, as many readers already know, I have designed my own line of supplements, the Forward Plus Daily Regimen, which are used at the Whitaker Wellness Institute. (Information on how you can purchase them and all the other supplements discussed in this book in the Resources section.) However, I am presenting the supplement plan in generic terms with the appropriate doses so that you can obtain them from whatever source you find most economical and convenient.

Your Supplement Shopping List

1. Cover all your bases and take a high-tech, high-potency multivitamin.

The first item on your shopping list is a *high-potency* multivitamin. Some of you may already be taking a multivitamin, but a multivitamin is not necessarily a high-potency multivitamin, which is essential. Unlike the outmoded multivitamins of the past, high-tech, high-potency multivitamins contain higher doses of essential vitamins and minerals than are called for by the RDAs. About two dozen of the essential vitamins and minerals that we need daily are available in any number of high-quality, high-potency multivitamins. There is only one mineral that you don't want in a multivitamin: iron. High levels of iron have been linked to an increased risk of heart disease, and unless you have been diagnosed as having iron deficiency, you should not take it.

There are several good brands of multivitamins to choose from, but only a few come close to what I think should be in a high-potency multivitamin. I recommend these brands: Maxi Life Powder (Twin Labs); Perfect Hardcore Pak (Nature's Best); Opti-Pack (Supernutrition); Multi Nutrient Pak (Schiff), and Multi-Nutrients (Ethical Nutrients.) You should be able to find at least one of these—if not all—at your local health food store or pharmacy.

Please note that I recommend higher doses of vitamin C (2,500 milligrams daily) and E (800 milligrams daily) than are in most multivitamins. The label will show how much of a specific vitamin is in each multivitamin. If a multivitamin has some but not enough of these or other vitamins I recommend, you can take additional doses of those particular supplements.

2. Supplement your multivitamin.

The next items on your shopping list are the *additional* supplements on the Age Loss ODAs that probably will not be found in most multivitamins or will not be in the correct doses. Also, I recommend several additional supplements, including The Energizers, and the one Muscle Builder that I have already described. These supplements are now available at virtually every health food store. In all likelihood you will have to buy them individually, but you won't have any trouble finding them: Each label will be clearly marked with the names listed below.

Supplements:

Antioxidants	Daily Dosage
Vitamin C	If necessary, add additional vitamin C supplements to your multivitamin to reach 2,500 milligrams daily.
Vitamin E	If necessary, add additional vitamin E supplements to your supplement multivitamin to reach 800 milligrams daily.
Ginkgo biloba	Take two 60-milligram capsules. (Look for standardized extract of 24 percent ginkgoflavone glycosides.)

Essential Fatty Acids

Omega-3 fatty acids	Take two 1,000-milligram softgel capsules. (The label should specify that two 1,000-milligram capsules equal 360 milligrams EPA and 240 milligrams DHA.)

The Energizers

Chromium picolinate	Take two (100 micrograms each).
Coenzyme Q10	Take two (30 milligrams each).

Lipoic acid	Take two (25 milligrams each).
Potassium-Magnesium-Aspartate	Take two (500-milligram) capsules.
Green Drinks	Mix three teaspoons in water or juice and drink on an empty stomach.

3. Special Rx for Weeks One to Four Only: Creatine Monohydrate, the Muscle Builder

One additional supplement not listed on the chart is creatine monohydrate. For the first four weeks that you are on the Age Loss Program, I recommend that you take creatine monohydrate to enhance your muscle strength. It is sold in a powdered form that can be mixed with water or juice. Begin by taking a large dose to build up a creatine reservoir in your muscles. For the first five days, take one heaping teaspoon (5,000 milligrams) of creatine monohydrate twice daily in juice or water. After that, take a maintenance dose of one teaspoon daily.

The reason I don't recommend creatine for the full ten weeks is that it is comparatively expensive. Since it is also very effective, I believe that taking it for four weeks will be enough for most of you. If you want to continue on creatine for the full ten weeks, that's fine.

4. DHEA: The Hormone for Health

Dehydroepiandrosterone (DHEA) is a natural hormone produced in the brain, skin, and adrenal glands. As we age, our levels of DHEA drop so that by around forty-five we produce only *half* of the DHEA we produced at twenty.

Many physicians and researchers—myself included—believe that the drop in DHEA is responsible in large part for the physical and mental decline that we have long associated with "normal" aging. That is why I believe it is of critical importance to restore DHEA to youthful levels in people who have low DHEA levels. Although DHEA supplements are available without a prescription, I do not recommend them for everyone. If you are under forty-five, you are probably making enough DHEA on your own. However, I do urge people over forty-five to get their DHEA levels checked by their doctor, and if they are low, then DHEA supplements are recommended.

Hundreds of studies have documented the vital role that DHEA plays in the body, particularly for immune function. As we get older, our immune system weakens, and this makes us more vulnerable to infections, cancer, and even autoimmune diseases such as rheumatoid arthritis. DHEA can *reverse* many of the problems that arise in immune function as we age. In a recent study conducted by Dr. Omid Khorram, a professor of medicine at the University of San Diego, nine healthy older men were given DHEA supplements for five months. Dr. Khorram found that DHEA stimulated the production of immune cells which fight against viruses and bacteria, as well as important cells called natural killer cells which help weed out cancerous cells before they can grow. Many patients have told me that since they have started taking DHEA, they rarely get sick and get far fewer colds and flus. If they do get sick, they recover much more quickly.

In addition to making people healthier, DHEA can also make people happier. In a recent study conducted at the University of San Diego researchers gave DHEA supplements to thirteen men and seventeen women, ages forty to seventy, for three months. For another three months the group received a placebo. During the time they were taking the DHEA, the researchers reported a "remarkable increase in perceived physical and psychological well-being for both men and women." The men and women not only felt better on DHEA but said they were better able to cope with stress.

Other studies have documented that low levels of DHEA increase the risk of heart disease in men. And interestingly, in one study of men over the age of forty, low levels of DHEA were strongly correlated with sexual dysfunction problems.

For all these reasons, I recommend having your DHEA levels checked by your doctor and supplementing DHEA if you need to. The usual dose is 50 to 100 milligrams daily for men and 25 to 50 milligrams daily for women. (If you have a history of prostate cancer, I do not advise that you use DHEA. There is absolutely no evidence that DHEA is harmful, but since it is a hormone, theoretically it may stimulate the growth of hormone-dependent cancers.)

HOW TO TAKE YOUR SUPPLEMENTS

Divide Your Dose High-potency multivitamins are different from the traditional one-a-day vitamins with which many of us grew up. These new high-tech multivitamins are meant to be absorbed throughout the day and are usually in two doses. Dose requirements vary from brand to brand, so follow the instructions on the label.

It is also best to take your supplements in two doses, one in the morning, the other in the afternoon, and always with a meal or a snack to avoid an upset stomach. Your body uses supplements as it needs them, and in most cases it excretes what it doesn't use within a matter of hours. This is particularly true for antioxidants such as vitamin C. If you take your supplements once a day instead of twice, you are leaving yourself unprotected at vulnerable times. You must replenish essential supplements throughout the day to achieve the full benefits of the Age Loss Program.

Depending on how a particular supplement is sold, it may not always be possible to divide the daily dose precisely in half. Don't worry about it. If you take 1,500 milligrams of vitamin C in the morning and 1,000 milligrams later in the day, that's close enough.

Take after exercising For best results on days when you exercise, take your supplements immediately following your workout with your meal or snack, when your muscles are primed to soak up the nutrients they lost during the workout.

Organize your supplements At the Whitaker Wellness Institute we distribute supplements in small prepackaged plastic packets, each containing the correct dosage. I urge you to take a few minutes to set up your week's supply of prepackaged supplements. Take one bag of supplements each morning with breakfast and carry one bag with you to take with lunch or dinner. This way you will not have to count pills every day, and you will always have your supplements with you when you need them. By taking a few minutes each week you will save time each day, and you'll never have to worry about what to take. This system is simple and convenient, and your supplements are always at your fingertips.

My method of using supplements will jump-start the rejuvenation process and rev up your body. By the end of ten weeks you will feel a real difference in terms of strength and stamina, and you will see a real difference in how you look.

Now that you have a thorough understanding of the power of the supplements that I'd like you to take, you are ready to move on to Step 2, "Lose a Decade's Worth of Fat." Here you will learn how Age Loss cuisine can help melt away the years and restore youthful metabolic function without dieting, suffering, or starving.

Step 2

Lose a Decade's Worth of Fat

Restore your youthful metabolism
Shed those extra pounds and extra years
Lose up to ten pounds of fat

PICTURE YOUR BODY LIGHTER and leaner, liberated from those extra pounds that seemed to sneak up on you somehow, ounce by ounce, inch by inch, over the course of the past decade. Now I will show you how to make this image a reality. I will teach you a skill that I have taught to thousands of my patients: how to use food as a tool of rejuvenation. I will show you how you, too, can use the power of food to revitalize and reclaim your body.

Age Loss cuisine is based on the premise that eating the right food can put the brakes on aging, whereas eating the wrong food will accelerate it. The same forces that rob us of youth and vitality weigh us down with unwanted and unhealthy pounds.

The principles of the Age Loss food plan are powerful but fairly simple. I will show you how to incorporate this plan into your normal diet, one week at a time. Once you know the basics, you will be able to adapt the plan to suit your personal food preferences.

Age Loss cuisine will not only help you slim down and

tone up but will generate some very real and positive changes in your physical and mental health. Based on the experiences of our patients, we know that by the time you have completed the full ten weeks, you will be *measurably* healthier. You will have more energy than you've had in years, and you will feel focused and more alert. And best of all, you will not—I repeat, *not*—feel hungry.

Ten Pounds of Fat per Decade

Most people are alarmed to discover that beginning at age forty, the average person gains about ten pounds of fat every decade. Worse, most of us are completely unaware of how and why those extra pounds creep up on us.

Over and over my patients tell me, "I used to be able to eat everything I wanted without gaining weight. Now I only have to look at food and I put on weight." Sound familiar? Rest assured, you are in good company. You are feeling the effects of a "midlife energy crisis," a slowdown in metabolism that is responsible for many of the problems that we have come to associate with "normal" aging.

Don't assume, however, that this weight gain is natural and therefore healthy. We vastly accelerate our metabolic slowdown by eating the wrong foods. Even in this nutritionally conscious day and age when many people believe they are eating wisely, most are subsisting on a nutrient-poor, low-quality diet that promotes aging and is responsible for that we-just-can't-do-what-we-used-to feeling.

It's painfully ironic to note that although one-third of Americans are seriously overweight (and food here is plentiful), most of us are nutrient starved. The effects of this form of malnutrition—including fatigue, loss of muscle tone, heart disease, and diabetes—are often not apparent until we hit middle age. At that point, too many people regard the effects as inevitable, figuring that they're just growing old and the deterioration "goes with the territory."

This is nonsense! The deterioration does not have to take place at all. There are things we can do to prevent it from taking hold and to alleviate it once it has. One of the most important ways is to eat sensibly, with the help of this program.

Age Loss cuisine has been designed with the help of Idel Kelly, our talented chef at the Whitaker Wellness Institute who has been giving our patients healthy and delicious meals for years. In fact, most patients incorporate this food plan into their diet at home. To make it easy for you to follow the plan, we've included at the end of this section many of our chef's favorite menus and recipes.

I promise that Age Loss cuisine will not leave you unsatisfied, unhappy, bored, or exhausted. Nor will you experience any of the unpleasant side effects often caused by low-calorie, low-nutrient diets, such as indigestion, constipation, depression, dry skin, and dry hair. On Age Loss cuisine your body will work the way nature intended it to, and this will be reflected in how you feel and how you look. Your hair will shine, your skin will glow with good health, your spirits will soar, and you will watch those extra years—and extra fat pounds—melt away.

Over the next ten weeks you will be eating hearty servings of many of the same foods that you already enjoy, and you will learn to enjoy some new foods as well. The primary difference is that the food you eat will be prepared without some of the unnecessary and harmful stuff—the "bad" fats, refined sugar, salt, and chemical additives—that add nothing but take away a great deal.

During Week One of the food plan, you will begin to make simple but highly effective changes in your diet. Each week you will phase in another important dietary change. By the end of ten weeks these small changes will add up to a significant loss in fat pounds and a significant gain in health.

I designed the program to accommodate people who prefer to make gradual changes. If you are so inclined, however, you can follow the entire program from Week One. Do whatever is most convenient for you.

AGE SAVER: Cook Your Food as "Cleanly" as Possible

Poach, steam, bake, or broil food. Do not cook in oil: This not only adds unwanted fat but promotes the formation of free radicals, which will promote "rapid aging." Instead, use nonstick cookware or a vegetable-based cooking spray, such as PAM, for cooking. After cooking, you can add a small amount of olive oil or sesame oil for flavoring.

WEEK ONE

Drink Eight Glasses of Water a Day

Drinking enough water is one of the easiest yet most effective ways to rejuvenate your body. Water is absolutely essential for maintaining the mineral balance that keeps our cells working well and our bodies functioning normally. As we age, we lose our water content, and in a sense, aging is a form of slow dehydration.

To prevent dehydration that can accelerate aging, I recommend that you drink eight glasses of water a day. Drink one glass when you get up in the morning, and one to two glasses half an hour before each meal. (Don't forget: You will already be drinking a glass of water each time you take your supplements. That accounts for two more.) And, as always, drink water after you exercise, frequently in hot weather, or anytime you feel dehydrated. One word of caution: Chlorine and other chemicals or contaminants such as lead often find their way into tap water. I therefore recommend drinking bottled water or investing in a water purification system for your home. The initial cost of the system may be several hundred dollars, but it is worth every penny.

Double Up on Your Veggies

If you're like most people, you are not eating enough vegetables. Therefore, beginning this week, I want you to concentrate on getting more fresh vegetables—and a greater variety —into your life. Vegetables are packed with vitamins, minerals, and phytochemicals, disease-fighting compounds which have powerful antioxidant activity that can slow down the aging process. Deep green leafy vegetables such as broccoli and kale have phytochemicals that are different from those of orange and yellow fruits and vegetables, such as cantaloupe, lemons, and winter squash. You need to eat a full assortment of different types of vegetables to get the full antioxidant protection that nature intended. Vegetables are also an excellent source of fiber, the food substance found in plants that is absorbed by the body and is essential for normal digestion. A low intake of fiber has been linked to cancer, heart disease, and many other health problems.

Please do not add unnecessary calories to your vegetables by slathering them with butter, margarine, or cream sauce. It is far better to season them with a sprinkle of lemon juice or dried or fresh herbs such as dill or basil.

Ideally, you should eat between five and eight servings of different vegetables every day. (Each serving should be at least half a cup.) If you think about it, that is a lot of food and a lot of healthy vitamins, minerals, and phytochemicals—items I am willing to bet you are very low in. In order to make room on your plate for your vegetables, you will probably have to cut back on your meat portion. That's precisely what I have in mind, as you will see in Week Three.

WEEK TWO

Eat Rejuvenating Carbohydrates

There are three kinds of nutrients: carbohydrate, protein, and fat. We need to eat a diet that provides an optimal balance of these nutrients. Carbohydrate is a general term for a wide range of foods, vegetables, fruits, cereals, grains, and legumes. Carbohydrates are an excellent source of energy. *Between 60 and 70 percent of your daily food intake should be in some form of carbohydrate.*

Protein is found in meat, fish, dairy, and plant foods such as beans. Protein is essential to build, maintain, and repair body tissue. *About 15 to 20 percent of your daily food intake should be in some form of protein.*

Fat is found in meat, dairy products, nuts, and oils. It is essential for energy and hormone production. *About 15 percent of your daily food intake should be in some form of fat.*

This week I want you to focus on eating the right kind of carbohydrates. There are two types of carbohydrates: complex and simple, or refined. Some carbohydrates accelerate the aging process. Some are powerful rejuvenators. Understanding the difference between the two types is the key to restoring youthful metabolism.

Simple carbohydrates are age *accelerators.* They include sugary snack foods, "junk" food such as potato chips, white bread, white rice, white pasta, presweetened breakfast cereals, snack foods, and most cookies and cakes.

The problem with simple carbohydrates is that they break down very rapidly in the bloodstream, causing a sharp rise in our blood sugar levels. These foods can actually cause a greater surge in blood sugar than that resulting from eating sugar straight from the box!

Eating these "bad" carbohydrates can wreak havoc on our metabolism. These foods can cause surges in blood sugar that not only exacerbate the problem of insulin resistance but also cause food cravings and constant hunger. This often leads to eating more "bad" carbohydrates, causing the cycle to repeat. Eating simple carbohydrates will put on extra weight and age us before our time.

Complex carbohydrates are *rejuvenators*. These include the following:

- Fruits and vegetables
- Whole-grain, unrefined products such as multigrain breads and cereals
- Pastas made from whole wheat or vegetable flours
- Beans such as lentils, black beans, and navy beans.

Although complex carbohydrates are good for us, they are not all the same, and we must limit the amounts we eat. With few exceptions, most breads and cereals ("starchy" foods) tend to cause a sharper rise in blood sugar than do vegetables. Eating too much of these foods can result in a sugar "crash," leaving you feeling hungry and depleted. To avoid the sugar highs and lows, limit servings of bread, cereal, and pasta to no more than three or four a day. (One serving is equal to one slice of bread, one cup of rice or pasta, or one cup of cereal.)

Starchy vegetables such as corn and potatoes should also be eaten in limited quantities. Limit servings of potatoes and corn to no more than two to three a week. (One serving equals one medium potato or one ear of fresh corn.) Although potatoes and corn are basically healthy and contain important vitamins and minerals, they, too, are broken down very rapidly and can cause a sudden blood sugar surge.

From Week Two on, eliminate white bread, sugary breakfast foods, snack foods, and junk food completely from your life—or at least until you finish the ten-week program! Replace them with whole grains. Seven- or nine-grain breads that are sold in most supermarkets are good choices. Rye or pumpernickel bread and crackers are also fine.

Rid your pantry of presweetened ready-to-eat breakfast cereals and switch to unsweetened cereals made from unprocessed grains. Oatmeal, rye flakes, barley flakes, and 100 percent bran flakes are good choices. I also provide a wonderful recipe (on page 86) for a delicious homemade granola that won't send your blood sugar spiraling.

I also recommend that you try breads made with sprouted grains because they are broken down by the body at a slower and steadier pace than breads made with flour and are often easier to digest. Sprouted breads, rolls, and even bagels are sold at health food stores and supermarkets, such as those made by Shiloh Farms, Food for Life, and Alvarado Street Bakery. Remember, these breads are not made with preservatives and must be refrigerated.

Eat Three Servings of Fruit Every Day

Fruit is a truly *rejuvenating* carbohydrate, and most of us do not eat enough of it. Similar to vegetables, fresh fruit is packed with wonderful vitamins, minerals, and phytochemicals that protect against disease. It is also a terrific source of fiber. A piece of fruit makes an excellent snack because it is refreshing, filling, and can satisfy a sweet craving. From Week Two on, I'd like you to eat three to four servings of fruit a day. (One serving is equal to one medium-size apple, pear, or orange, or about one cup of fresh sliced fruit.) Eat a piece of fruit when you feel hungry or compelled to reach for that cookie or candy bar!

WEEK THREE

Escape the "If It's Dinner, It Must Be Meat" Syndrome

This week I would like you to concentrate on cutting back on meat. When most of us think of protein, we usually think of meat, eggs, or dairy products such as milk and cheese, but in reality many plant foods are rich in protein. Raw nuts, beans, and some grains are all excellent sources of protein.

Americans eat about twice as much protein as their bodies actually need. The problem is that the type of protein most of us are eating does us more harm than good. The major source of protein in the American diet is red meat, a food that I personally believe humans were never intended to eat—and certainly not in the vast quantities that we do.

Red meat is loaded with saturated fat, which is converted to cholesterol in your body; this raises blood cholesterol levels and increases the risk of heart disease, stroke, colon cancer, and gallbladder disease. By now you may have guessed that I don't eat red meat, and I advise you not to, either, at least during the rest of the time you are on the Age Loss Program.

Don't worry, I'm not asking you to live on sprouts. You can still enjoy hearty meals of fresh fish and lean poultry. The fish or poultry portion should occupy no more than one-third of a standard-size dinner plate; the rest of the plate can be filled with complex carbohydrates.

I don't expect you to eat fish or poultry every day, and in truth I would like you to give other protein sources a try. On page 79 there is a menu and recipes that include hardy and delicious meatless meals. Some of my favorites include home-made Hardy Winter Bean Soup, Vegetarian Lasagna, and Vegetable Tostado. Make a special point of trying at least one of these recipes this week, and at least for the next seven weeks try to cut out red meat from your diet altogether.

WEEK FOUR

Go Organic

This week I would like you to begin to eat foods that are as close to their natural state as possible—in other words, food that has not been stripped of its micronutrients and fiber (roughage) or pumped full of salt, sugar, artificial sweeteners, flavorings, stabilizers, and preservatives. I highly recommend organically grown food, which is not polluted by insecticides, covered in wax, or adulterated in other ways. Organic produce is also better from a nutritional standpoint, since it is grown under conditions that preserve the vitamin and mineral content of the soil. Even if you eat organic food only for the duration of the time you are on the program, you will be giving your liver a much-needed rest. The liver is responsible for detoxifying every potentially harmful chemical that enters your body. Given the toxic environment that we live in, it is one of the most overworked of all our organs. Reducing the toxic load can give your liver time to rejuvenate with the rest of your body.

Whether or not the produce you use is organic, it still needs to be thoroughly rinsed before being eaten. (Even organic produce can pick up germs during handling.) Produce that is not organic should also be rinsed and peeled, especially if it is the kind of fruit or vegetable that is routinely waxed, such as apples, peppers, and cucumbers. The wax literally seals the pesticides to the skin.

I also recommend that you eat free-range or organic poultry if possible. Organic or free-range poultry is raised humanely on wholesome feed, without hormones, antibiotics, or other pollutants. Granted, organic poultry is a bit more expensive, but think of it as an investment. You are paying for the chemicals to be removed from your food. Many supermarkets carry organic poultry. If you can't find it, you can order it by mail from one of the purveyors listed in the Resource section at the end of this book.

WEEK FIVE

Discover the Joy of Soy

This week I want you to learn about a food that is lacking in the diet of most Americans: soybeans.

If there ever was a perfect food, it is the soybean. And if there ever was a food that can rejuvenate your body, it is one made from soybeans. (I have some *great* news for you. Soy is also a wonderful tool for revitalizing your sex life. See page 182 for more information.) It so happens that soybeans contain a very high quality protein that is every bit as good as meat protein, and in my opinion better.

Soybeans are packed with protein, are chock-full of good phytochemicals, and contain absolutely no saturated fat. They are also incredibly versatile. Soybeans can be made into a milk, turned into tofu (which can be used instead of meat or cheese in many recipes), pulverized into protein powder that can be made into a healthful beverage, texturized into a product that can be used as a substitute for chopped meat, or made into a thick paste called miso, which cooks into a tasty soup. I like to eat soybeans lightly steamed in their natural form, and they are a favorite snack at the Whitaker Wellness Institute.

Ironically, the United States is the world's leading producer of soybeans but not the world's leading consumer. Much of our soybean crop is shipped to Japan and other Asian countries where soybeans are a dietary staple. American women are four times more likely to die from breast cancer than are Japanese women, and American men are five times more likely to die from prostate cancer than are Japanese men! One reason is soy. Soy is rich in hormonelike compounds called isoflavones (which include genistein, daidzein, and biochanin A) that are similar to the hormones produced by the body. There is one important difference, however; isoflavones found in soy normalize hormone levels in the body and stop the growth of hormone-dependent cancers.

Soy milk Soy milk is quite delicious and comes in an array of flavors. There are even some prepackaged soy milk shakes that not only taste good but are excellent sources of isoflavones, something dairy milk shakes are not. I use soy milk instead of cow's milk on my cereal, and believe me, you can't tell the difference.

Veggie burgers A new crop of soy-based vegetarian burgers has appeared. You will find them on the frozen food shelves of your neighborhood supermarket. My personal favorite is the Boca Burger, which comes preseasoned and has an amazingly good flavor that will put you in mind of your favorite fast-food hamburger. I'm not kidding. Boca Burgers can be panbroiled or microwaved, which makes them convenient to use. Served with tomato, onion, and a spot of ketchup or mustard on a whole-grain roll, they make a wonderful burger substitute and are an excellent source of isoflavones.

Tofu Tofu has a mild flavor which literally soaks up the taste of any food or flavoring that is added to it. Tofu can be blended with fruit to make a creamy shake or used instead of cheese or meat in a vegetarian lasagna. It can even be grilled on the barbecue with barbecue sauce. In China, tofu is called "the meat without bones" because it is used interchangeably with meat. (You will find a terrific tofu recipe on page 109.)

(Not all soy products are the same. Some soy products are so overly processed that they do not contain beneficial isoflavones. These include soy sauce and soy-based ice cream, which you should avoid.)

WEEK SIX

Get the Right Fat into Your Life

This week I would like you to incorporate more good fat into your diet. Although you need to trim the "bad" fat from your diet, some forms of fat are essential for life. These "good" fats are appropriately called essential fatty acids.

There are two types of essential fatty acids: omega-6 and omega-3. Omega-6 fatty acids are found in nuts, seeds, avocados, grains, and most cooking oils. Most people get adequate amounts of omega-6 fatty acids through their diet.

Omega-3 oils are generally found in cold-water fatty fish, deep green vegetables, and some grains and seeds. Our hunter-gatherer ancestors had a ratio of omega-6 to omega-3 fatty acids of about five to one. Today, the ratio is around twenty-four to one, and many researchers believe that the decline in omega-3 fatty acids is contributing to the high rates of heart disease and cancer. This shortage is due to the fact that it is difficult to get enough omega-3 fatty acids from food alone. Even if you eat a lot of fatty fish, omega-3 fatty acids are very fragile and can be destroyed by heating. In addition, much of the omega-3 fatty acids are concentrated in and under the skin of fish, which is often discarded prior to cooking. That is why I recommend that everyone take fish oil capsules as part of the Age Loss Program's supplement plan. But now you can also obtain omega-3 fatty acids with flaxseed oil, an excellent dietary source. Flaxseed contains more omega-3 fatty acids than fatty fish, as well as high amounts of lignans, a phytochemical that neutralizes harmful hormones that stimulate the growth of breast and prostate cancer. Flaxseed oil can also be purchased at health food stores (in the refrigerated section) or by mail, and it makes an excellent salad dressing. Try to consume two tablespoons of flaxseed oil daily. (See the recipe on page 95.) Fresh flaxseed can be purchased at health food stores and ground in a coffee grinder for a smoother consistency. Sprinkle about one-fourth cup of freshly ground flaxseed on hot or cold cereal for a wonderful source of omega-3 fatty acids. (On days that you don't have flaxseed oil, I recommend that you have one-fourth cup of fresh flaxseed.)

WEEK SEVEN

Learn About the Benefits of Phytochemicals

This week I would like to reinforce the importance of eating a wide variety of fruits and vegetables. By now you are eating five to eight servings of fresh vegetables and three to four servings of fresh fruit every day. You are undoubtedly feeling years lighter already! As mentioned earlier, fruits and vegetables are packed with phytochemicals, substances that fight disease and promote age loss. Here is a list of the most important phytochemicals and a description of foods that contain them. Whenever possible, try to incorporate these important phytochemicals into your daily food plan.

Allicin (and other sulfur compounds) Crushed garlic releases pungent sulfur compounds, including allicin, that can lower blood cholesterol and fight the formation of cancerous tumors. These compounds can also help prevent infectious diseases, including colds and flu. Legend has it that during the Middle Ages, monks ate huge quantities of garlic to ward off the plague.

Ellagic acid Cherries and strawberries are loaded with ellagic acid, which is a natural anticancer compound, and they are also delicious sources of vitamins.

Liminoid Found in the essential oils of orange and other citrus fruit peels (and the white pulp between segments) as well as in dill, caraway, and lemongrass, liminoid inhibits the formation and reduces the size of tumors in animals. It is now being tested on breast cancer patients.

Lutein This phytochemical is a member of the carotenoid family. Studies show that people who eat a large amount of lutein-rich foods are much less likely to develop macular degeneration, the leading cause of blindness in older people. Lutein is found in deep green leafy vegetables such as kale and collard greens.

Lycopene A tomato a day may keep prostate cancer away. In a six-year study of more than forty-eight thousand men, Harvard researchers found that those who ate tomatoes, tomato sauce, or pizza more than twice a week reduced their risk of developing prostate cancer by about 30 percent. Why? Researchers credit lycopene, the chemical that makes tomatoes red and that is a powerful antioxidant. Cooked tomatoes seem to offer more protection than raw tomatoes, and lycopene works better when combined with a small amount of fat. (See my recipes for Pizza and Vegetarian Lasagna, which are high in lycopene.)

Quercetin Red and yellow onions are a rich source of quercetin, a remarkable phytochemical that is a natural anti-inflammatory and also protects against heart disease and some forms of cancer. Studies have shown that the more onions we eat, the lower our risk of stomach cancer and heart attack.

Sulforaphane Found in broccoli, brussels sprouts, cabbage, and kale, this phytochemical stimulates the production of enzymes in the body that disarm free radicals before they can harm healthy cells. Eat one serving of these foods daily.

Xanthophyll This carotenoid, found in spinach and collard greens, appears to protect against age-related macular degeneration.

Zeaxanthin Found in green leafy vegetables, this antioxidant is also found in the macula of the eye and is believed to help preserve good vision.

Many of these phytochemical-rich foods are incorporated in the recipes that begin on page 86. Try to use them in your menus whenever you can.

WEEK EIGHT

Fiber Awareness Week

Another type of food that most Americans do not get enough of is fiber. This week I want you to be aware of good sources of fiber so that you can eat them on a regular basis.

There are two types of fiber: soluble and insoluble. Soluble fiber, which is found in foods such as apples, oat bran, and broccoli, can lower blood cholesterol levels. Insoluble fiber, which is found in wheat bran, beans, and celery, speeds up the movement of food through the intestine and can prevent constipation and other digestive problems. Fiber does not provide any calories or nutrients and yet is critically important in preventing insulin resistance, the condition that can throw your metabolism out of whack and promote accelerated aging. Fiber can also help prevent other serious illnesses, including colon cancer and heart disease. Unfortunately, fiber is often stripped away during food processing, and few Americans eat enough fiber in their daily diets. In fact, most Americans eat only half of the 30 grams a day of fiber that they should be eating.

Another important function of fiber is that it slows the breakdown of carbohydrates in the blood, preventing those sudden spikes in blood sugar that I have been talking about. Fiber is also rich in the mineral magnesium, which protects against diabetes, and phytic acid, a phytochemical that may also have a role in regulating sugar. However fiber performs its magic, the net result is that it helps control blood sugar levels and prevent insulin resistance.

According to a recent study, fiber may be the single most important foodstuff in combating insulin resistance. As part of the Nurses' Health Study, Harvard researchers tracked the diets of 65,173 women for six years. After analyzing food diaries kept by the women themselves, the researchers found

71

that women who ate a "starchy" diet, drank sugary soft drinks, and ate the least amount of fiber had two and a half times the rate of Type II diabetes, which as we've seen is caused by insulin resistance. In other words, eating too much of the wrong kind of carbohydrate and too little fiber is a recipe for insulin resistance, diabetes, and premature aging. If you follow Age Loss cuisine and eat the right kind of carbohydrates and enough fiber, you will achieve age loss.

WEEK NINE

Try New Grains

Most of us are in a food rut. We tend to eat the same foods every day and rarely try anything new. I am convinced that many people overeat out of sheer boredom with the food they are eating. No matter how much they eat, they are not satisfied because their taste buds crave excitement. Eating a wide variety of foods and trying new foods will help prevent the kind of mealtime boredom that leads to bingeing, which is as unhealthy as it is satisfying.

One of the goals of Age Loss cuisine is to get you out of the "food rut" by introducing you to new foods. I would now like to introduce you to two new grains that I have recently discovered: amaranth and quinoa. I use the word "new" advisedly because these grains have been around for centuries but are being rediscovered by health-conscious people because of their unique properties. What these grains have that others such as wheat do not is high amounts of protein, which helps to prevent carbohydrate-induced sugar highs.

Amaranth This grain was a staple among the Aztecs more than five hundred years ago. It is a small seed with a mild, nutty flavor that resembles sesame. Unlike most other grains, amaranth is rich in lysine, one of the eight essential amino acids that the body cannot produce itself; this makes it an excellent protein source. Amaranth can be eaten as a side dish like rice (it's actually quite good with soy sauce) or used in baking. It is sold in supermarkets and health food stores. (See page 106 for a recipe for Spicy Moroccan Amaranth.)

Quinoa Although used as a grain, quinoa is actually a dried fruit of a plant that is native to Bolivia and Peru. The Incas called quinoa the "mother grain" and considered it sacred because they believed it promoted health and longevity. They knew intuitively what nutritionists have only recently discovered: Quinoa is a rich, high-quality source of protein, the kind normally found in meat and dairy products. When used as a grain, quinoa has a light, fluffy texture that makes it a pleasant substitute for potatoes and rice. Quinoa flour, which is becoming more popular, can be used for baking and is a wonderful alternative for people who are allergic to wheat flour. Quinoa is sold in both supermarkets and health food stores.

WEEK TEN

Keep Going

Now that you have begun your last week on the Age Loss Program, you should be eating a greater variety of healthy food than you have eaten in your entire life. You have added fruits and vegetables to your diet, trimmed the bad fat, increased the good fat, and are eating the right kind of protein and carbohydrates.

The good things that you are putting into your body are now showing on the outside. You look trimmer, lighter, and healthier. You feel more alert and energetic. By following the Age Loss food plan, you have taken a giant step toward achieving the ultimate goal of shedding ten years in ten weeks.

Over the past ten weeks you have made some positive changes in your diet. I urge you to incorporate them into your life permanently. It will help you maintain the youthful advantage you have already gained.

AGE SAVER: To Rejuvenate Your Metabolism, Eat After You Exercise

If you are on a regular exercise regimen, particularly one that causes you to sweat or elevates your pulse for any significant length of time (twenty minutes or more), it is best to take in high-quality nutrients within thirty to thirty-five minutes after exercising. That's when your muscles are depleted of the vital nutrients they lost during the workout and are primed to soak up energy. It is more likely that the nutrients will be used to replenish hardworking muscle cells than be diverted to fat cells.

AGE LOSS CUISINE IN ACTION

Now that you understand why some foods promote aging and some prevent it, you are ready to put this knowledge into action. The following pages contain some general guidelines in terms of acceptable beverages, snacks, and occasional desserts that can be included in your food plan. I also provide a sample menu that you can follow for one week, as well as delicious recipes that have become favorites of mine and my patients.

Acceptable Beverages

In Week One, I told you to begin drinking eight glasses of water a day. Obviously, water should be your primary beverage, but you are allowed to drink other beverages, too.

Coffee As you undoubtedly know, coffee contains caffeine, a mild stimulant. That is why it provides that lift in the morning and why it and other caffeinated products should be avoided at night. Although health gurus preach that coffee is unhealthy, this teaching is based on old studies that have since been refuted. New research indicates that moderate coffee drinkers do not seem to be at any risk, so I believe that a cup of coffee every day is perfectly fine. (If you put cream in your coffee, however, I urge you to switch to low-fat or skim milk because cream is loaded with saturated fat. And please do not use sugar or artificial sweeteners.)

Green Tea I also recommend one cup of tea a day, preferably green tea, which is more lightly processed than the black tea common in America and retains more of its important phytochemicals. Studies have shown that compounds found in green tea can protect against cancer, especially lung cancer. In a study conducted at the American Health Foundation, mice were exposed to nitrosamines, a potent cancer-causing agent. Half of the exposed mice were given green tea in their drinking water, and the other half were not. The results were really quite remarkable: There were 45 percent fewer cases of lung cancer among the tea-drinking mice. And studies in Japan have shown that people who live in regions where green tea is produced and who, we can assume, drink a lot of it have significantly lower rates of cancer than any other group of people in Japan.

By the way, green tea also contains "catechins," which

are compounds that have antibacterial properties. They are effective against streptococcus mutans, the bacteria responsible for tooth decay and gum disease.

Keep in mind that green tea contains about half the caffeine of a cup of coffee, so don't drink it too close to bedtime. Herbal teas (peppermint, chamomile) are also allowed.

Spirits Under the Age Loss Program's food plan, you can also enjoy an occasional glass of wine or beer. Ales and wines have been part of our diet for thousands of years, and they have long been valued for their medicinal properties. In fact, the Talmud teaches that "wine is the foremost of all medicines." Studies have shown that moderate drinking of wine (less than two glasses daily) can reduce the risk of heart disease and stroke. Keep in mind, however, that alcohol is fattening. So don't overdo it. In addition, don't drink it if you have a history of hypoglycemia, liver disease or alcoholism, or are taking any medication that should not be taken with alcohol. Although I am certain that I don't have to remind you of this, I will anyway because the message is so very important: Never drink and drive.

Milk Many people have difficulty digesting milk, and it is also the cause of numerous allergies, so I do not recommend it wholeheartedly for everyone. If milk agrees with you, stick to skim or low-fat for at least these ten weeks and drink it in moderation. Some people may worry that they will not get enough calcium if they don't drink milk. Plain, nonfat yogurt is an excellent source of calcium and is easier to digest than plain milk. It can be mixed with raw nuts and fruit for a quick breakfast or lunch. Green leafy vegetables are also a wonderful source of calcium, so if you follow Age Loss cuisine (and take your multivitamin, which should include between 1,000 and

1,500 milligrams of calcium), you will get all the calcium you need.

Foods to Avoid

Processed meats There are some foods that I regard as unfit for human consumption, and they are banned from the Age Loss Program. Processed meats (hotdogs, salami, bologna) are high on the list. These foods are laden with saturated fat (the worst kind) and chemicals such as nitrites, which are converted in the stomach into potentially carcinogenic chemicals called nitrosamines. Nitrosamines promote the formation of free radicals, and people who routinely eat foods high in nitrites have higher rates of gastrointestinal cancers. Think of it this way: Eating processed meat is the equivalent of eating a plateful of free radicals. In recent years low-fat versions of luncheon meats made from chicken and turkey (instead of the usual pork and beef) have become popular and are being promoted as healthy foods. Although they are low in fat, which is good, they still contain nitrites. Therefore, I can't recommend them.

A truly delicious sausage that I can wholeheartedly recommend is chicken sausage, which can be found in gourmet shops, health food stores, and better supermarkets. These sausages are not smoked (which promotes nitrosamine formation), are low in fat, and do not contain preservatives. Instead, they are seasoned with fresh basil, pine nuts, or sun-dried tomatoes, which gives them a unique flavor. They are not only a healthier alternative but I believe they actually taste better than traditional sausage. Get out of the food rut and try some!

Margarine One kind of fat that isn't essential and I would like to see it banished from your diet forever is margarine. At one time margarine was touted as good for your heart because it does not contain any saturated fat, but we now know that the process which turns oil into margarine can promote the formation of trans-fatty acids in the body; these can actually raise blood cholesterol levels and may even increase the risk of breast cancer. For most people an occasional small pat of butter is a lot healthier than margarine. (If you have abnormally high blood cholesterol, you should avoid butter and margarine altogether.)

Roasted nuts, seeds, and nut butters When nuts are roasted, they become oxidized and loaded with free radicals. I therefore recommend that you eat only raw nuts and seeds, which can be purchased from health food stores. Almonds, pumpkin seeds, and sunflower seeds are good choices. It is also advisable to avoid peanut butter since it is made with roasted nuts and undergoes a process that can promote the formation of trans-fatty acids. You can, however, eat nut butters made with raw nuts, such as almond butter or tahini (made from sesame seeds) that can be purchased at health food stores. They are both healthy and so delicious that I promise you won't even miss peanut butter.

Artificial eggs Those strange chemical-laden artificial "egg-like" products are discouraged, but real eggs are permitted on Age Loss Program cuisine and so are frozen prepackaged egg whites. Eggs are high in cholesterol, however, concentrated in the yoke. We get around this problem by recommending that you blend one egg yolk with three egg whites. Mixed with vegetables and served with salsa, this makes a terrific breakfast omelette. It is one of my favorite breakfasts.

AGE LOSS CUISINE AT A GLANCE

A Guide to Daily Eating

On the pages that follow, I provide a week's worth of daily menus and a variety of recipes. One of the advantages of this food plan is that you can devise your own meals and menus simply by using this chart as a guideline.

CARBOHYDRATES

Starches and Grains
3–4 servings from the following choices:
Bread, cereal, pasta, or cooked grains
(1 serving = 1 slice of bread, 1 sprouted bagel, or 1 cup of cooked cereal, pasta, or cooked grains)

Vegetables
5–8 servings of any kind of vegetables (but corn and potatoes are to be limited to twice a week apiece)
(1 serving = 1/2 cup cooked or 1 cup raw)

Fruit
3–4 servings of any kind of fruit
(1 serving = 1 medium-size whole fruit or 1/2 cup sliced fruit)

PROTEIN

3–4 servings from the following choices:

Fish, poultry, and tofu
1 serving = 4–6 ounces, or about the size of a deck of cards

Beans
1 serving = $^1/_2$ cup cooked

Soy milk
1 serving = 1 cup

Raw nuts and seeds
1 serving = 2 tablespoons raw nuts, seeds, or raw nut butter

Yogurt and cottage cheese
1 serving = 1 cup

Eggs
1 serving = 1 egg yolk mixed with three egg whites (limit to twice a week)

FAT

Limit fat intake to 2 tablespoons of flaxseed oil (preferred) or olive oil (use only occasionally)

Making the Age Loss Cuisine Work for You

By now you should have a pretty good idea of which foods are potent rejuvenators and which will make you age faster than you need to. Many of you will already be able to devise your own meals based on what you have learned. To get you started, however, we have provided a week's worth of sample menus and some wonderful recipes so that you can see how easy it is to eat well and still shed those extra years.

Sample Menus

Monday

Breakfast
Easy homemade granola (^{1}/$_2$ cup), topped with 1 cup of plain yogurt or flavored soy milk, fresh berries, orange and peach slices (see recipe on page 86)
Small sprouted bagel (preferably with no butter)
Coffee or tea with low-fat milk

Lunch
Boca burger on whole-grain bun with dark green lettuce, sliced tomato, sliced red onion, and sprouts
Sesame Mandarin Coleslaw (see recipe on page 88)
1 fresh apple
Herbal or green tea

Dinner
Grilled chicken over Spicy Moroccan Amaranth (see recipes on pages 106–107)
^{1}/$_2$ cup of blueberries and strawberries over ^{1}/$_2$ cup of frozen nonfat yogurt
Herbal tea

Tuesday

Breakfast
1 cup of hot cereal (such as steel-cut oats, old-fashioned oats, oat groats, wheat berries, or barley) made with 1 cup of flavored soy milk
^{1}/$_4$ cantaloupe with ^{1}/$_2$ cup of nonfat cottage cheese and sliced kiwi
Coffee or tea with low-fat milk

Lunch
Chicken salad (4–6 ounces of white meat chunks mixed
with 1/2 apple, diced, avocado slices, and 2 tablespoons
of no-fat salad dressing)
6 small rye crackers
Herbal or green tea

Dinner
Homemade pizza (see recipe on page 91)
Mixed green salad with low-fat dressing
1 fresh orange
Herbal tea

WEDNESDAY

Breakfast
Whole-grain pancakes
Cold sliced fresh peaches
Coffee or tea with low-fat milk

Lunch
Whole wheat pita stuffed with humus (see recipe on page
104), cucumber, sliced tomatoes, sprouts, shredded
dark green lettuce, and 1/2 sliced avocado
Broccoli, tomato, and red onion salad with low-fat dressing
Herbal or green tea

Dinner
Grilled chicken with brown rice and mushroom teriyaki
sauce (see recipe on page 99)
Mixed green salad with flaxseed dressing (see recipe on
page 95.)
1 cup fresh fruit cup (1/2 apple cut in chunks, 1/2 sliced
banana, and 1/4 cup berries of choice)
Herbal tea

THURSDAY

Breakfast

1 cup of bran flakes with $1/2$ cup of soy milk or low-fat
milk
1 cup of plain yogurt with $1/4$ cup of sliced banana
Coffee or tea with low-fat milk

Lunch

Homemade hardy winter bean soup (see recipe on page
93)
Greek salad (dark greens with artichoke hearts, feta
cheese, black olives, cucumbers, and tomato; see recipe
on page 102)
Olive oil and balsamic vinegar dressing
6 small rye crackers
1 fresh peach, orange, or pear
Herbal or green tea

Dinner

Vegetarian lasagna (see recipe on page 90)
Butter lettuce, radicchio, and fresh grapefruit segments
with flaxseed oil dressing
Nonfat frozen yogurt with cooked blueberries

FRIDAY

Breakfast

1 cup of hot oatmeal topped with cinnamon and $1/4$ cup of
sliced bananas
$1/2$ grapefruit
Coffee or tea with low-fat milk

Lunch

Grilled vegetable sandwich (grilled mushrooms and eggplant slices seasoned with fresh basil and 2 tablespoons feta cheese on sprouted bread with dijon mustard)

Three-bean salad (see recipe on page 97)

One fresh fruit, any kind

Herbal or green tea

Dinner

Asparagus and leek tart (see recipe on page 98)

Cucumber salad (see recipe on page 87)

Spiced pears (see recipe on page 96)

Herbal tea

SATURDAY

Breakfast

2 slices of French toast made with sprouted or whole-grain bread (see recipe on page 103)

1 cup of yogurt with ½ cup of fresh berries

Coffee or tea with low-fat milk

Lunch

1 cup of vegetable chili (see recipe on page 100)

Tossed green salad with low-fat dressing

½ canteloupe

Herbal tea

Dinner

Grilled salmon with dill sauce (see recipe on page 101)

Spiced couscous (see recipe on page 94)

Fresh greens with flaxseed oil dressing

Easy fruit crisp (see recipe on page 89)

Herbal tea

SUNDAY

Breakfast

Assorted fresh vegetable omelette (1 egg yolk mixed with
3 egg whites)
1 slice of rye toast, preferably with no butter
$^1/_2$ grapefruit
Coffee or tea with low-fat milk

Lunch

Vegetable tostado (see recipe on page 105)
Herbal or green tea

Dinner

Tofu teriyaki (see recipe on page 109)
1 cup of brown rice
Mixed green salad with flaxseed oil dressing
$^1/_2$ cup of fruit sorbet topped with strawberry slices
Herbal tea

EASY HOMEMADE GRANOLA

Serves 4

2 cups rolled oats
1 teaspoon ground cinnamon
$^1/_4$ cup chopped walnuts or almonds
$^1/_4$ cup sunflower seeds
$^1/_4$ cup or less walnut oil
$^1/_4$ cup brown rice syrup or honey

1. Preheat the oven to 350° F.
2. In a large bowl, combine the oats, cinnamon, walnuts, seeds, oil, and honey. Use your hands to mix well and distribute the oil and honey evenly throughout the mixture.
3. Place the mixture on a cookie sheet and toast for 10 to 15 minutes, turning frequently with a spoon when the cereal is browned on top. Be careful not to let the mixture burn.

NOTE: Feel free to substitute any other grain, nuts, or seeds.

CUCUMBER SALAD

Serves 2

1 cucumber, peeled and thinly sliced
$1/4$ cup rice vinegar
1 teaspoon sesame seeds, toasted
$1/2$ teaspoon chopped fresh ginger
1 teaspoon brown rice syrup

1. Combine all ingredients
2. Chill for 2 hours.
3. Remove the ginger before serving. Use a mesh tea ball for the ginger for easy removal.

SESAME MANDARIN COLESLAW

Serves 6

Dressing

$^1/_4$ cup low-sodium soy sauce
$^1/_4$ cup sesame oil
2 tablespoons rice vinegar
2 teaspoons spicy mustard
$^1/_2$ teaspoon grated fresh ginger
1 teaspoon brown rice syrup

1 medium head green cabbage
4 carrots
1 small can mandarin oranges, drained

Garnish: toasted sesame seeds

1. Combine all the dressing ingredients, then set aside.
2. Shred the cabbage and carrots in a food processor, or by hand.
3. Mix the dressing with the shredded cabbage and carrots.
4. Add the mandarin oranges and top with the toasted sesame seeds.

EASY FRUIT CRISP

Serves 4

2 cups fresh fruit (peaches, blueberries, apples, etc.),
    peeled if necessary and cut into small chunks
$1/4$ cup apple juice concentrate
$1/4$ cup whole wheat flour
$1/2$ cup uncooked oatmeal
2 teaspoons ground cinnamon
2 teaspoons walnut or extra-virgin olive oil
$1/4$ cup chopped walnuts
2 teaspoons honey
1 tablespoon brown rice syrup

1. Preheat the oven to 350° F.
2. Layer the chopped fruit in the bottom of an 8- by 8-inch nonstick baking dish. Pour the apple juice concentrate over the fruit.
3. Combine the flour, oatmeal, cinnamon, oil, and walnuts.
4. Sprinkle the oatmeal mixture over the fruit. Drizzle with the honey and brown rice syrup.
5. Bake for 30 to 40 minutes, or until the oatmeal is browned.

VEGETARIAN LASAGNE

Serves 8

Marinara Sauce

3 cloves garlic, minced
Pinch of oregano
2 tablespoons chopped fresh Italian parsley
2 tablespoons chopped fresh basil
6 to 8 mushrooms, sliced
1 green bell pepper, chopped
$^1/_2$ yellow onion, chopped
8 ripe tomatoes, peeled and chopped, or 2 large
    (28-ounce) cans of whole tomatoes

1 zucchini, finely chopped
1 yellow squash, finely chopped
1 carrot, finely chopped
$^1/_4$ teaspoon ground nutmeg, or to taste
2 pounds fat free ricotta cheese
2 pounds lasagna noodles

1. Mix all the ingredients for the marinara sauce and simmer for 20 minutes.
2. Preheat the oven to 350° F.
3. Mix all the chopped vegetables with the nutmeg and ricotta cheese. Cover until ready to use.
4. Cook the noodles according to the package directions.
5. In a large rectangular pan arrange one layer of noodles, then one layer of the vegetable-cheese mixture. Continue to alternate layers until all ingredients are used.
6. Bake for 45 minutes.
7. Top with the marinara sauce before serving.

HOMEMADE PIZZA

Serves 6–8

Crust

1 package active dry yeast
1/2 cup warm water (105° to 115° F.)
3/4 cup all-purpose flour
3/4 cup whole wheat flour
2 tablespoons olive oil

Toppings

1/2 teaspoon olive oil
1/2 teaspoon balsamic vinegar
1 clove garlic, chopped
2 plum tomatoes, chopped
1/4 cup chopped fresh basil
1 1/2 cups fresh spinach
1/4 cup thinly sliced red onion
1 teaspoon grated Parmesan cheese

1. Dissolve the yeast in the warm water in a medium-size bowl.
2. Combine the flours and 1 tablespoon olive oil in a separate bowl. Add to the yeast and stir well.
3. Turn out on a lightly floured board. Knead until smooth and elastic, about 6 to 8 minutes.
4. Lightly grease a bowl. Place the dough in the bowl and turn once to grease the surface. Cover and let rise until double in size, about 1 1/2 hours.

5. While the dough is rising, prepare the toppings. Heat all the vegetables in a nonstick saucepan for 2 to 3 minutes, just to wilt them. Drain the juice from the vegetables.
6. Preheat the oven to 400° F.
7. When the dough has doubled in size, punch it down and roll out into a 12-inch circle.
8. Place on a round pizza pan and brush lightly with remaining oil. Let rise for 10 minutes, then bake for 10 minutes.
9. Lightly brush oil on the baked crust.
10. Add the toppings and Parmesan, and bake for 10 minutes.

HARDY WINTER BEAN SOUP

Serves 6

1 (14-ounce) can low-sodium, defatted chicken or
   vegetable stock
1 (28-ounce) can whole tomatoes, mashed
1 medium red potato, finely chopped
1 medium white turnip, finely chopped
1 whole serrano chile or $\frac{1}{2}$ teaspoon crushed red
   pepper
$\frac{1}{2}$ teaspoon black pepper
1 leek (white part only), sliced
$\frac{1}{2}$ bunch Swiss chard (green part only), finely
   chopped
$\frac{1}{4}$ yellow onion, chopped
1 clove garlic, chopped
2 teaspoons olive oil
1 (19-ounce) can white beans (kidney beans, Great
   Northern, etc.)
$\frac{1}{2}$ cup barley

1. In a large stockpot, place the stock, tomatoes, potato, turnip, whole chile, and black pepper. Bring to a boil, lower the heat, and simmer for 20 to 25 minutes, until the chopped potato is soft.
2. In a large sauté pan, place the leek, Swiss chard, onion, garlic, and then the oil (so as not to burn the oil). Sauté for 3 to 4 minutes, until soft.
3. Add the sautéed vegetables to the soup and simmer for 20 minutes. Add the beans and barley, and cook for 10 more minutes.

SPICED COUSCOUS

Serves 4

2 cups water
1$\frac{1}{2}$ tablespoons olive oil
$\frac{1}{2}$ teaspoon curry powder
$\frac{1}{4}$ cup frozen peas
6 ounces plain couscous

1. Bring the water to a boil. Add the oil, curry, and frozen peas.
2. Pour over the couscous, cover, and let stand for 10 minutes. Fluff the mixture with a fork and then serve.

FLAXSEED OIL DRESSING

$\frac{1}{2}$ cup flaxseed oil
$\frac{1}{4}$ cup tarragon vinegar
$\frac{1}{2}$ tablespoon chopped fresh parsley
1 clove garlic, chopped
$\frac{1}{2}$ tablespoon chopped chives

1. Combine all ingredients in a medium bowl. Blend well with a wooden spoon.
2. Store in a covered jar in the refrigerator. Shake well before using. (One serving is 2 tablespoons.) Can be stored for one to two days.

SPICED PEARS

Serves 2

2 Bartlett pears, peeled, cored, and halved
$1/2$ cup apple juice concentrate
2 cups water
3 or 4 whole cinnamon sticks
3 or 4 whole cloves
1 teaspoon almond extract

Sauce

$1/4$ cup Amaretto
2 teaspoons cornstarch dissolved in 2 teaspoons cold
    water

Garnish: sliced almonds (toasted 4 to 5 minutes in
    the oven) and bittersweet chocolate shavings

1. Preheat the oven to 400° F.
2. Combine the pears, apple juice concentrate, water, cinnamon sticks, cloves, and almond extract in a small baking dish. Cover with a lid or aluminum foil and bake for 1 hour.
3. Remove the pears with a slotted spoon and place in individual serving bowls. Reserve the juice for the sauce.
4. Prepare the sauce: Combine the Amaretto and the baking juice in a saucepan. Bring to a boil to burn off the alcohol. Add the cornstarch mixture to the sauce. Stir until thickened.
5. Pour some sauce over each pear and sprinkle with the almonds and chocolate.

THREE-BEAN SALAD

Serves 6–8

1 cup pinto beans, cooked
1 cup black beans, cooked
1 cup garbanzo beans (chickpeas), cooked
2 cloves garlic, chopped
1 red bell pepper, chopped
$1/4$ cup chopped black olives
$1/2$ cup fat-free Italian dressing

Combine all ingredients and chill before serving.

ASPARAGUS AND LEEK TART

Serves 6

1/2 cup plain bread crumbs
Olive oil
8 ounces asparagus, trimmed and cut into 2-inch
    pieces
2 leeks (white part only), sliced
2 tablespoons flour
2 cups frozen (*or* 8 fresh) lightly beaten egg whites
1 cup fat-free ricotta cheese
1/4 cup shredded low-fat, low-sodium Swiss cheese
    (Alpine Lace)
1/2 cup skim milk
1/4 teaspoon ground nutmeg

1. Preheat the oven to 425° F.
2. Mix the bread crumbs with 1 tablespoon of oil until moistened. Pat into a large pie dish and toast in the oven for 5 to 6 minutes. Let cool.
3. Blanch the asparagus in boiling water for 2 to 3 minutes. Drain and set aside.
4. In a medium sauté pan over medium heat, place the leeks and then 1 tablespoon of oil (so as not to burn the oil). Cook for 4 to 5 minutes. Sprinkle with flour, stir to coat, and transfer the mixture to a bowl.
5. Add the eggs, ricotta cheese, Swiss cheese, milk, and nutmeg. Mix well. Pour over the toasted bread crumbs in the pie dish.
6. Bake until puffy and brown, about 40 minutes. Let stand 10 minutes before slicing.

GRILLED CHICKEN WITH BROWN RICE AND MUSHROOM TERIYAKI SAUCE

Serves 2

2 boneless chicken breasts (4 to 6 ounces each)
$^1/_4$ cup low-sodium soy sauce
$^3/_4$ cup water
1 tablespoon apple juice concentrate or brown rice
    syrup
$^1/_2$ teaspoon rice vinegar
2 cups sliced mushrooms
Garlic to taste
1 cup cooked brown rice

1. Grill the chicken breasts.
2. While the chicken is grilling, simmer the soy sauce, water, apple juice concentrate, vinegar, mushrooms, and garlic in a saucepan for about 15 minutes.
3. Pour this mixture over the chicken and brown rice.

VEGETABLE CHILI

Serves 4

2 (29-ounce) cans no-salt whole tomatoes, mashed
4 cups cooked pinto beans
$^1/_2$ cup chopped onion
$^1/_2$ cup chopped bell pepper
2 to 4 tablespoons chile powder, or to taste

Garnish: sliced green onions

1. In a saucepan, mix the tomatoes, beans, onion, bell pepper, and chile powder.
2. Cook for 45 minutes, adding water as needed.
3. Garnish with the green onions.

GRILLED SALMON WITH DILL SAUCE

Serves 2

2 salmon fillets, 4 ounces each
$^1/_2$ cup plain nonfat yogurt
$^1/_2$ teaspoon chopped fresh dill

1. Preheat the oven to 350° F.
2. Grill the salmon about 5 minutes on each side. Place in a baking dish, cover, and bake for 10 to 15 minutes to replace the moisture.
3. Combine the yogurt and dill. Chill.
4. Serve the sauce over the salmon.

GREEK SALAD

Serves 6

4 ounces "baby green" lettuce mixture
3 cucumbers, peeled and diced
$^1/_2$ purple onion, thinly sliced
3 tomatoes, chopped
1 cup artichoke hearts, packed in water
$^1/_4$ cup chopped fresh basil
1 cup no-fat Italian dressing
1 tablespoon feta cheese

Mix all the ingredients and let marinate in the refrigerator at least 2 hours.

FRENCH TOAST

Serves 6

8 egg whites
$^1/_2$ cup skim milk
$^1/_2$ teaspoon vanilla extract
Ground cinnamon to taste
12 slices whole wheat bread

Garnish: fruit-juice-sweetened jam, *real* maple syrup,
    raw honey, applesauce, or your favorite no-sugar,
    no-fat topping

1. Mix the egg whites, milk, vanilla, and cinnamon in a bowl.
2. Dip each slice of bread in the egg mixture.
3. Cook on a nonstick griddle, turning, until brown on both sides.
4. Serve with your choice of garnish.

HUMMUS SANDWICHES

Serves 2

2 cups cooked garbanzo beans (chickpeas)
$1/4$ cup tahini (sesame butter)
2 cloves garlic, minced, or to taste
Juice from $1/2$ small lemon, or to taste
1 teaspoon finely chopped fresh parsley

1. Place all the ingredients except the parsley in a food processor and puree until smooth. If dry, add a little skim milk.
2. Stir in the parsley
3. Serve as a sandwich filling on pita or whole-grain bread with lettuce and tomato slices.

VEGETABLE TOSTADA

Serves 6

6 cups cooked pinto beans
$1/2$ cup salsa (hotness to your preference)
6 whole wheat tortillas
$1^{1}/_{2}$ cups chopped onions
1 head iceberg lettuce, shredded
2 carrots, shredded
$1^{1}/_{2}$ cups chopped green bell pepper
$1^{1}/_{2}$ cups chopped tomatoes
6 teaspoons nonfat plain yogurt

1. Preheat the oven to 300° F.
2. Puree the pinto beans in a food processor with the salsa. Place in a nonstick baking dish and bake for 30 minutes.
3. Warm the tortillas for a few minutes in the oven. Keep warm and moist in a tortilla warmer or wrapped in a warm kitchen towel.
4. Place the beans, vegetables, yogurt, and salsa in separate bowls so that each diner may spread a tortilla with the toppings.

SPICY MOROCCAN AMARANTH

Serves 6

1 cup cubed eggplant
Garlic-flavored nonstick vegetable cooking spray
1 large onion, chopped
1 clove garlic, chopped
1 red pepper, chopped
1 green pepper, chopped
4 carrots, thinly sliced
1 zucchini, cut in $1/2$-inch slices
1 yellow summer squash, cut in $1/2$-inch slices
1 cup kidney beans, rinsed and drained
$1^1/2$ cups tomato sauce, preferably low salt
$1^1/2$ cups low-salt, fat-free vegetable broth
$1/2$ cup raisins
2 teaspoons curry powder
$1/4$ teaspoon cayenne pepper
1 teaspoon paprika
1 cup amaranth (see Note)
3 cups cold water

1. Drain the eggplant cubes on a paper towel for 10 minutes.
2. Spray a large, heavy skillet with the cooking spray. Sauté the onion and garlic until translucent, about 5 minutes.
3. Add the red and green peppers, carrots, and eggplant. Sauté for 10 minutes, stirring occasionally.
4. Add the zucchini and squash. Cook for 2 more minutes.
5. Add the beans, tomato sauce, broth, raisins, curry powder, cayenne, and paprika. Cover, bring to a boil, then simmer for 20 minutes.

6. Bring the amaranth and water to a boil in a saucepan with a lid. Lower the heat and simmer for 25 minutes. The grains will absorb the water and bind together.
7. Spread the amaranth on a platter and top with the vegetables.

NOTE: After trying amaranth plain, try cooking it with a hint of herbs, spices, or other seasonings, Garlic, oregano, chopped fresh basil, black pepper, parsley, and rosemary are a few suggestions.

Contributed by Judith Eaton, New York Nutrition Network.

GRILLED CHICKEN

Serves 2

2 skinless, boneless chicken breasts
    (4 ounces each)
Juice from 1 fresh lemon
1/8 teaspoon fresh pepper
2 cloves garlic, finely chopped
2 tablespoons chopped parsley

1. Marinate the chicken breasts overnight in the lemon juice, pepper, garlic, and parsley. Turn once after several hours.
2. Grill the chicken until cooked through or bake in a single layer in a nonstick baking dish at 350° F. for 45 minutes.

Contributed by Judith Eaton, New York Nutrition Network.

TOFU TERIYAKI WITH SPICY ORANGE GLAZE

Serves 6

2 pounds extra-firm tofu
½ cup low-sodium tamari sauce
½ cup brown sugar
2 teaspoons vegetable oil
2 cloves garlic, minced
1 teaspoon minced fresh ginger
2 tablespoons vinegar
2 tablespoons honey
¼ cup orange juice
Dash of dry sherry
Ground pepper to taste
1 (8-ounce) can water chestnuts, sliced

1. Drain and pat the tofu dry. Slice each block into 8 slices.
2. Combine the tamari, brown sugar, oil, garlic, ginger, vinegar, honey, orange juice, sherry, and pepper to use as a marinade.
3. Pour half of the marinade into a 9- by 13-inch ovenproof glass baking dish. Arrange the tofu cutlets over the marinade. Sprinkle the water chestnuts over each cutlet
4. Cover the tofu and water chestnuts with the remaining marinade. Let stand for several hours or more.
5. When ready to serve, remove the tofu and water chestnuts from the marinade and braise in a little of the marinade about 3 minutes on each side, until brown.
6. Serve the tofu with rice and snap peas (frozen are fine).

Contributed by Judith Eaton, New York Nutrition Network.

Step 3

⌀

SHED TEN YEARS' WORTH OF FINE LINES AND WRINKLES

Restore youthful radiance and glow

Slow down and reverse skin aging

Protect against sun damage

My skin used to be one of my best features. I always used to get compliments on my skin. Since my mid forties, my skin has become dull and blotchy. The antioxidant creams that Dr. Whitaker recommended gave me back my peaches and cream complexion. I like what I see in the mirror.

ROSEMARY W., 47

My skin hasn't looked so good since I was a teenager.

CLAIRE G., 51

OVER THE PAST DECADE your skin has undergone many changes, and if you're like most folks, you're probably not happy about a lot of them. Let me begin by telling you some news that will put a smile on your face. If you follow my Age Loss Program, your skin will not only look dramatically better but you will actually reverse much of the damage that your skin has suffered over the past ten years. Thanks to recent breakthroughs in skin care technology, you can restore a youthful tone and quality to your skin and make a very positive difference in how well (and how good) you look. And the best part is that it won't take you more than minutes a day.

I will show you how to make optimum use of the new generation of high-tech over-the-counter skin care products that are available from drug and department stores, skin salons, neighborhood health food stores, and mail-order catalogs. Although all these products are available without a prescription, some are sold only at skin salons or by physicians. I will explain which of these new products really work, why they work, and where to buy them.

At the Whitaker Wellness Institute, we follow the Age Loss Program's skin care regimen which was designed with the help of noted dermatologist Richard E. Fitzpatrick, founder of Dermatology Associates of San Diego County, and a specialist in skin rejuvenation. (Although I will be recommending products from several different skin care lines, you may be interested in purchasing the same products that we use at the Institute. See page 265 for more information.)

You may wonder why a physician who is neither a dermatologist nor a plastic surgeon is so concerned about such a "cosmetic" problem as skin care. Indeed, some of you may feel we should simply accept wrinkled, sagging skin gracefully because it is an inevitable part of growing older.

To me this is utter nonsense. Given the choice of seeing a glowing, youthful face or a dull, wrinkled face when looking into a mirror, I know what I would choose, and now the choice is yours. By following this easy plan, you will see a noticeable difference by the end of ten weeks, I guarantee it. I do not take this position because I worship at the altar of wrinkle-free skin. But I am as concerned about the basic health and quality of your skin as I am about any other organ or system in your body, and for good reason.

As explained earlier, we must take care of ourselves from the outside in as well as from the inside out. Beauty is not, as the saying goes, only skin deep. On the contrary, the condition of our skin and how we look on the outside is actually a good barometer of what is going on inside our body. Far from being an opaque screen that conceals, our skin is actually a window that reveals. What it reveals tells us a lot about our general health.

Skin, you see, is vulnerable to the same forces that cause the aging of our internal organs and systems. For reasons I will explain, premature wrinkling, discoloration, "sun spots," and other external signs of aging may actually be warning signs that we are aging on the inside as well. In fact, every step of my Age Loss Program will have a beneficial effect on your skin.

Skin is not a decoration or just a container. Skin is the largest organ system in the body and one of the hardest working. In addition to its obvious role in providing cover and protection for our internal organs, skin performs many other critical tasks. Skin is our first line of defense against viruses, bacteria, fungi, and other foreign and toxic substances. Skin is also essential for maintaining body temperature and enables us to retain fluids, such as blood and water, which are essential for life. It plays an important role as well in the operation of the endocrine system, which is responsible for producing the hormones that govern all our bodily functions. Finally, skin is instrumental in the production and storage of vitamin D, which is essential for the absorption of calcium. Needless to say, if we don't take care of our skin, we are hurting ourselves more than we realize.

How Skin Ages

Skin is the only organ that is constantly exposed to the environment, and because of this it pays a steep price in terms of wear and tear.

Skin consists of two layers. The outer layer—the one we can see—is the epidermis, and the inner layer is the dermis. Underneath the skin lies a subcutaneous layer of fatty tissue that separates our skin from our muscles and bones.

Did you ever wonder why younger skin tends to look pink and fresh, whereas older skin tends to have a sallow, worn-out appearance? One reason is that as we age, we do not make new cells as quickly or as efficiently. The epidermis contains mature cells that are ready to be shed. New skin cells are waiting in the wings to replace them. The older we get, the longer it takes for these new cells to replace the old cells. In other words, we are "wearing" our old, dull cells for a longer period of time, and it shows.

To prevent this we need to understand what essential elements we lose as we age. Then we need to replenish these elements (as you will do for the next ten weeks).

We lose collagen The dermis is made up mainly of collagen, the tissue which provides the scaffolding that supports the outer layer of cells, the epidermis. As we get older we experience a sharp decline in collagen production, and this literally pulls the support out from under the top layer of skin.

Think of collagen as a mattress and the skin as a sheet that covers it. If the mattress were to shrink and become lumpy, the sheet would sag and wrinkle. That is basically what happens to our skin when we lose collagen.

We lose water Another reason that young skin looks plump and supple is that it is filled with water. As we get older we

113

lose cells that help the skin retain moisture; in fact, skin loses about 30 percent of its water content. As a result, our skin becomes drier.

We lose hormones Finally, there is a significant midlife decline in the production of key hormones, and this, too, adversely affects skin quality. Hormones such as estrogen and testosterone help the skin retain moisture, and when production of these hormones diminishes, skin dries out and wrinkles become more apparent.

AGE SAVER: Get Your Beauty Sleep

When you don't get enough sleep, you will not only feel tired but you will *look* tired. While you are sleeping, your pituitary gland releases growth hormone and other growth factors that stimulate the production of new collagen, which is necessary for cell repair and renewal. And that's not all. If you don't get enough sleep, you get dark circles under your eyes because the skin around your eyes loses its elasticity and moisture content when you are tired. This affects the way light is reflected off this area, producing the illusion of dark shadows.

SUN DAMAGE: THE MAIN CULPRIT

The vast majority of our skin problems, including so-called laugh lines, crow's-feet, and wrinkles, are due to what dermatologists call "photo aging," or damage caused by exposure to the ultraviolet (UV) rays produced by the sun. Compare the condition of the skin on your face to the condition of the skin on any other part of your body that is usually covered by clothing. The difference is striking. The skin that has rarely seen the light of day will look decades younger. UV light is the reason.

Damage from UV light is cumulative and can take years before it is apparent. Generally, by the time we reach our mid-thirties the long-term effects of UV exposure start to become visible in the form of fine lines, wrinkles, and telltale changes in skin tone and color. No one is immune.

Don't assume just because you are not a regular sun bather or you don't spend a lot of time at the pool or on the tennis court that you are safe. Most of us get a heavy dose of UV rays when we are going about our daily business, even when we are going to and from work or the grocery store. Over a lifetime this kind of brief but chronic exposure leaves its mark.

There are two types of ultraviolet rays: UVA and UVB. Both types stimulate the formation of free radicals on the skin. These free radicals are the very same highly reactive oxygen molecules that promote aging inside the body and are causative factors in such diseases as diabetes commonly associated with aging. (By the way, if you smoke cigarettes, you are essentially inhaling thousands of free radicals with each puff. By age forty smokers tend to have wrinkles comparable to people ten years older.)

UVB rays, commonly referred to as the burning rays, inflict immediate damage on the epidermis. Even brief exposure to UVB rays can turn sensitive skin red and cause pain and inflammation. UVB rays are particularly nasty because, in addition to promoting the formation of free radicals, they give off intense heat that actually "cooks" the DNA in the nuclei of skin cells. This causes genetic changes that can lead to serious problems, including skin cancer. All the antioxidants in the world can't protect you against the wrath of UVB rays.

UVA rays do not usually cause perceptible reddening of

the epidermis. Rather, UVA rays inflict their damage by injuring the cells of the dermis and the subcutaneous layer of fat that are underneath the outer layer. This causes the kind of hidden damage that shows up years later as lines and wrinkles, and sometimes even as skin cancer.

The full effect of UV exposure is not immediately apparent. Our bodies' own antioxidant defense network deactivates some free radicals before they can inflict harm. But as you know, our antioxidant levels decline as we age. To compound the problem, numerous studies have documented that even a small amount of UV light—not even enough to give a blush to the skin—causes a steep drop in antioxidant levels. In other words, every time you expose your face to the sun, your skin is being robbed of the antioxidants that protect it and keep it healthy and young looking.

Cosmetic changes to skin are the most innocuous effects of UV exposure. Skin cancer can be deadly. One million new cases of skin cancer are diagnosed each year in the United States. That number is expected to grow, especially as baby boomers age. Baby boomers grew up in an era when leisure time was abundant, sunbathing was fashionable, and a suntan was considered a sign of good health. Remember those advertisements for suntan lotions which boasted that the products filtered out the "bad" burning rays but allowed in the "good" tanning rays? Today we know that there is no such thing as a "good" tan. We know that a tan is not a sign of health but is instead a sign that skin has been injured.

UV damage does not stop at the skin's surface; its effects are felt well beneath it. In fact, exposure to UV radiation can severely weaken the immune system's ability to fend off viruses and bacteria and to halt the growth of malignant tumors. This proves once again how neglecting one organ system can have a profound impact on another and how by fortifying one system you also exert a positive effect on the other.

UNDOING A DECADE'S WORTH OF DAMAGE, ONE DAY AT A TIME, A FEW MINUTES a DAY

The goal of the Age Loss Program's skin care regimen is not merely to hide damaged skin but to make our bodies act younger. In other words, we must fortify our skin to defend itself against the forces that promote aging. To do this we need to replenish what time has taken away.

As I outline my skin care regimen, I will tell you about products which do just that and how to choose the ones that are right for you. These products are designed to be used on the face, neck, and hands, the areas that are most exposed and therefore show the most signs of damage.

Although my skin care regimen is for both men and women, and for skin of all types, from time to time I will also make specific recommendations for particular skin problems (such as oily or dry skin) or especially sensitive skin.

Heal and Protect Damaged Skin

To rejuvenate your skin, you must first stimulate your body's natural repair mechanisms. But you cannot repair your skin if it is constantly being bombarded by UV rays and is therefore forced to expend its energy on defending against new wounds rather than healing old ones. I'm asking you to give your skin a ten-week vacation from the stress of normal wear and tear. To do so, for the next ten weeks you will need to wear as strong a sunscreen or sunblock as you possibly can every day on your face, neck, hands, and other exposed areas. Sunscreen filters out most of the dangerous rays, whereas sunblock prevents any UV rays from being absorbed by the skin. Even if you have a dark complexion and do not burn easily, you should still wear a sunscreen. Wearing a sunscreen will not only prevent further damage but will allow your skin to begin the healing process, and it will be tremendously therapeutic.

Studies show that if mildly sunburned skin is covered with sunblock, it will continue to repair itself even during subsequent exposure to the sun. The lesson is clear: The first step in restoring your skin to a more youthful condition is to protect it from additional UV damage.

So in addition to wearing a sunscreen or sunblock, for the next ten weeks try to avoid being outdoors for prolonged periods, especially during the peak burning hours of 10:00 A.M. to 3:00 P.M.

USE THE BEST SUNSCREEN

Be sure you choose your sunscreen carefully. All are not equally effective, and most do only half the job. For example, while sunscreens are fairly efficient at screening UVB rays, they are not particularly effective against UVA rays. Finding a sunscreen that protects against both is often difficult, mainly because it is not easy to tell by reading the label. In order to be sure that you are getting adequate UVA protection, look for products that contain a compound called avobenzene or Parsol 1789.

People with oily skin may find that Parsol 1789 makes their skin even more oily and prone to acne; they should therefore look for a sunscreen designed specifically for oily skin or use a sunblock.

People with dry to normal skin may find Parsol 1789 or other ingredients used in sunscreen somewhat irritating. For example, some people find PABA (para-aminobenzoic acid), a common sunscreen ingredient, irritating, which is why many sunscreens are advertised as PABA-free. The fact that a product is PABA-free, however, is no guarantee that other ingredients won't irritate you.

I strongly suggest that before applying any sunscreen (or

any skin care product, for that matter) to a sensitive area such as your face, you first test it on a small patch of skin on your upper arm, cover it with a Band-Aid, and leave it on for twenty-four hours. If there is no sign of irritation, you can use it on other parts of your body.

By the way, do not assume that a sunscreen that purports to be hypoallergenic will be problem-free, either. It is virtually impossible to design a skin care product that will be perfect for everyone. If you are being treated for a particular skin condition, ask your dermatologist for a recommendation or simply do the skin patch test to find the one that works best for you.

As many of you know, sunscreens are rated by SPF or sun protection factor. A sun protection factor of 15 would mean that if it normally takes a person ten minutes to burn, with an SPF of 15, he can stay out in the sun fifteen times longer before burning. You should wear a sunscreen with an SPF of at least 15.

Unfortunately, too many people assume this means you can go out into the sun for 150 minutes without worrying about damage. That is not the case. Remember, there are also UVA rays to worry about. UVA rays do not typically cause a burn, but they do cause serious long-term damage to the dermis and subcutaneous layers.

USE A SUNBLOCK

Another option is to use a *sunblock* that actually forms a physical barrier between your skin and UV rays. Using a sunblock is like wearing a T-shirt on your face. Sunblocks contain micronized titanium dioxide, and although they may be less irritating than sunscreens for some people, they are a bit more difficult to use because if not applied evenly, they can form white streaks.

Cosmetic companies have recently started including sunscreens in their moisturizers and foundations. Keep in mind that these products do not provide the same UVA protection as products containing Parsol 1789. And even if you use a combination sunscreen and foundation, you will still need a sunscreen on your hands, neck, and other exposed areas.

Here are my recommendations for good sunscreens and sunblocks, and how they can be obtained.

- Shade UVA-Guard Broad Spectrum Sunscreen Lotion with Parsol 1789. This sunscreen is sold at pharmacies and drug stores.
- Beaver-43. This waterproof sunblock has both UVA and UVB protection, and is sold primarily in sporting goods stores.
- Ti-silc Moist SPF 45. This sunblock is excellent for people who need strong protection; it is also easy to use. Available through physicians. For information call Humatech Labs at 1-800-593-SKIN.
- Sunshade Z-20 by Skinceuticals: This new sunblock is available through physicians or skin salons; can also be ordered by telephone. For information call 1-800-811-1660.

Restore the Antioxidant Balance

The antioxidant supplements that I recommended in Step 1 and the antioxidant-rich foods that I recommended in Step 2 will work on your skin from the inside. However, you can also attack the problem from the outside by using the new antioxidant skin creams that are just beginning to appear on the market.

Vitamin C Serum and Cream

Vitamin C serum and cream are the most exciting skin care breakthroughs to occur in decades. Why? Because these products really work, and not only that, they are wonderful for the health of your skin.

I recommend that you use a *high-potency* vitamin C serum or cream every morning. Women should apply it underneath their makeup and sunscreen. Men can use it before or after they shave, depending on their preference. A daily step-by-step skin care regimen is provided at the end of this chapter.

The vitamin C products that I recommend will make a real difference not only in the appearance but in the health and quality of your skin. Vitamin C serum and cream will also fortify and protect your skin against further UV damage from the sun.

Why does vitamin C serum and cream work better than simply taking oral vitamin C supplements? Vitamin C supplements and the vitamin C we obtain from food help maintain collagen to some degree, but only a small amount of the vitamin C we take orally gets into the skin. Delivering vitamin C directly to the skin is an elegant and efficient way to get this essential vitamin where it is needed. Once absorbed by the skin, vitamin C appears to stimulate the formation of new collagen, which is one of the ways it improves the appearance of skin. New collagen helps restore skin tone, plump up wrinkles, and fill in small lines, giving skin a more youthful look. Topically applied vitamin C improves blood supply to the skin, giving the skin a more youthful glow.

Vitamin C can minimize fine lines and reduce light wrinkles in the troublesome and noticeable areas around the mouth and eyes. Deeper furrows and wrinkles will not disappear but should show improvement. Vitamin C will also help improve skin color and tone, resulting in a more taut, less flabby look.

Finally, and most important, vitamin C has been shown to protect skin from damage inflicted by UV light and to reduce some of the inflammation caused by UV exposure. In fact, studies have shown that topically applied vitamin C can prevent one of the most dangerous effects of UV exposure: the suppression of the immune system. This means that vitamin C not only has a cosmetic effect but offers serious protection against further damage to the skin.

Vitamin C should be used only in specially formulated products designed specifically for external use. Otherwise, it will not be absorbed by the skin. Do not rub vitamin C from a pill or capsule directly onto the skin; it could be very irritating, not to mention totally ineffective. There are a number of vitamin C skin care products on the market and more debuting every month. Bear in mind that not all vitamin C products are alike, nor are they equally effective. Many of the cosmetics that purport to have vitamin C contain so little that they are useless, nor are they in a form that can easily be absorbed.

Vitamin C is available as a liquid serum or as a cream. Since potent vitamin C serums and creams may cause discomfort if they get into the eyes, weaker versions are designed for use around the delicate eye area.

The serums are stronger than the creams and are therefore more effective. People with very sensitive skin may find them to be too irritating, however, and may prefer to use a cream.

As of this writing, none of the vitamin C products listed below are sold in stores, but you can obtain them easily from the sources given. If you have age-related damage near your eyes, you should use a milder form around the eyes in addition to the stronger form on the rest of your skin.

- Cellex-C Skin High Potency Serum; Cellex-C Eye Contour Gel; Cellex-C Skin Firming Cream; Cellex-C Eye Contour Cream, from Cellex-C Cosmaceuticals, Inc. Available through physicians or skin salons; can also be ordered by telephone. For information call 1-800-903-4321.

- Topical Vitamin C High Potency Serum; topical Vitamin C Eye Gel from Skinceuticals. Available through physicians or skin salons; can also be ordered by telephone. For information call 1-800-811-1660.
- C-Esta Serum, C-Esta Cream, and C-Esta Eye Gel from Jan Marini Skin Research, Inc. Available through physicians and skin salons. For information call 1-800-347-2223.
- "Deep C" by Ecological Formulas. For information call 1-800-888-4585.

RETINOL CREAM

For more than a decade high-potency vitamin A creams have been available by prescription and used as antiwrinkle creams. The first vitamin A cream was tretinoin, better known as Retin-A, which was originally used as an acne treatment. Dermatologists who treated adults with Retin-A noticed that it wasn't just their acne that disappeared; very often fine lines and wrinkles would also vanish. Word got out about this amazing "wrinkle cure," and it soon became one of the most prescribed medications in the United States. More recently, another type of vitamin A cream, retinoic acid, marketed under Renova, became the first prescription wrinkle cream approved by the Food and Drug Administration (FDA). Although these prescription products work very well, the downside is that they can be irritating and can cause skin to redden and peel.

Here's some exciting news. As of this writing, a weaker cousin of retinoic acid, *retinol,* is being used in several new over-the-counter skin care products. Similar to Retin-A and Renova, retinol can help reduce fine lines and wrinkles, and reduce age-associated skin discolorations without troublesome side effects. Similar to vitamin C, retinol sloughs off old cells and stimulates the formation of new cells. Retinol is unique in that it can do something that vitamin C cannot: It can "reprogram" the new cells to act more like cells on youthful skin. The new cells not only look younger but retain moisture the way younger skin cells do. The best news is that since retinol is not as strong as the prescription vitamin A products, it is not nearly as irritating, although it may cause minor redness and some flaking in people with sensitive skin. I recommend that you use a retinol product as part of your evening skin care regimen.

Retinol products can be obtained through the following sources:

- AFIRM from TxSystems by Medicis Pharmaceutical Corporation. This product comes in three strengths: .15, .30, and .60. It is available through physicians. Check with your physician to see which strength is best for you. For information call 888-896-2100.
- Avon Retinol Recovery Complex PM Treatment. Available through Avon sales representatives. To place an order call 1-800-FOR-AVON.
- Healthy Skin Anti-Wrinkle Cream by Neutrogena Corp. This product is sold in pharmacies, drug stores, and department stores.
- Retinol-15 and Retinol-30 by Sothys, U.S.A., Inc. Available through skin salons and spas. This product comes in two strengths. Retinol-15 is weaker than Retinol-30. Check with your skin care professional to see which strength is best for you. To find a salon near you or to place an order, call 1-800-325-0503.

Alpha Hydroxy Acids: Stimulate the Growth of New Cells

If you want your skin to look smoother, brighter, and more youthful, you need first to slough off the old cells so that new cells can take their place. This process is called stimulating cell turnover.

Alpha hydroxy acids (AHAs) do just that. They stimulate

old cells to shed more rapidly, revealing younger, fresher-looking skin. Alpha hydroxy acids are substances found in fruit, sugar, wine, and milk. The most commonly used AHAs are lactic acid (from sour milk) and glycolic acid (from sugarcane). I recommend that you apply an AHA cream or lotion each night before you apply your retinol product. Although AHA skin care products are relatively new, AHAs have been used for centuries in one form or another. In fact, legend has it that Cleopatra took goat milk baths and that Marie Antoinette washed her face in wine. What these women and their ladies in waiting knew instinctively has since been proven scientifically: AHAs can penetrate the surface of the skin, "unglue" or "burn off" old cells, and stimulate new cell growth.

If used conscientiously, AHAs can give skin a fresher appearance and can reduce the appearance of fine lines and wrinkles. Unlike vitamin C cream, which stimulates collagen formation in the inner dermis, weak AHAs work primarily on the epidermis. AHAs can also increase the number of complex sugar molecules in the skin called glycoaminoglycans (GAGS), which help skin retain moisture. Although there have been few clinical studies on products that contain low concentrations of AHAs, you definitely can see a real difference in the skin quality of people who use them. Their skin typically looks fresher and more youthful.

Given the fact that there are so many AHA products, how do you select one that is right for you? The answer is to pick one that is not too weak and not too strong. I recommend that you choose a product that contains a concentration of AHAs between 8 and 10 percent. This is potent enough to make a real difference in your skin but not so strong as to cause irritation for most people.

If you have very sensitive skin, start by using a product that contains less than 5 percent AHAs. Any AHA over 5 percent may cause a mild stinging sensation (remember, you are applying acid), but it should disappear immediately.

Some manufacturers state the percentage of AHA right on the label, which makes choosing a product easier for consumers, but many do not. If you can't find a product that does list the percentage of AHA on the label, then read the label to make sure its AHA (such as glycolic or lactic acid) is situated high up on the list of ingredients—in the second or third spot. This means that it is one of the primary ingredients. If it isn't, chances are there is only a tiny amount of AHA in the product.

Before using any AHA, be sure to do the patch test on your arm to see if it causes an irritation. Repeat the test on a small spot on your face, and if all is well within twenty-four hours, then you can use it all over your face.

AHAs do many good things for your skin, but one of the bad things they do is make skin very sensitive to UV light. Therefore, if you use an AHA, you must use a sunscreen or sunblock every day. If you do not want to use a sunscreen or sunblock, do not use an AHA.

- Skin Smoothing Cream by Neostrata. Available from physicians and skin salons. Call 1-800-865-8667.
- Exuviance by Neostrata. A lower-strength AHA that is effective but good for sensitive skin. Available at department stores or by calling 1-800-234-8578.
- Murad Night Reform. Available from skin salons or by telephone. Call 1-800-33-MURAD.
- Murad Sensitive Skin Smoothing Cream. Available from skin salons or by telephone. Call 1-800-33-MURAD.
- Alpha Hydrox 10 percent AHA. Sold at drugstores.
- Ponds Age Defying Complex. Sold at drugstores and pharmacies.

Rehydrate Your Skin

From midlife on, our cells tend to lose their moisture content. This causes skin to become flatter and dryer, and facial lines and wrinkles to become more apparent. Dryness is a concern because it causes itching and flaking all over the body. The condition is not only uncomfortable but makes the skin more vulnerable to infection. Maintaining the proper moisture content of skin is therefore important. I have several recommendations for enhancing the moisture content of your skin.

1. Drink enough water. In Step 2 I urged you to drink eight glasses of water daily. Now I will give you another important reason to do so: Water helps replenish the moisture lost by the skin. This sounds ridiculously simple, but it is very important.

2. Cool down with water. Keep a spray container of water handy and spritz your skin with water several times daily to cool it down and restore lost moisture.

3. Use a moisturizer. Finally, you will need to use an external moisturizer on your face up to several times daily, depending on your skin type, to seal moisture in. Of all the skin care products I have discussed, a moisturizer will produce the most immediate results. Almost instantaneously a good moisturizer will smooth out fine lines and wrinkles, and plump up the skin, making these imperfections less noticeable. The problem with moisturizers is that their effects are very short-lived. *For maximum benefit they must be applied several times a day: morning, midday, and evening.* If you live or work in a very dry environment, you may need to reapply your moisturizer even more frequently.

There are numerous moisturizers on the market. The most effective ones contain either hyaluronic acid or essential fatty acids, preferably both. Hyaluronic acid is a compound found deep within the skin. It binds with water to prevent evaporation; in fact, it is one of the most potent water-holding compounds known.

Essential fatty acids seal moisture in the skin. A diet that is deficient in essential fatty acids will result in flaky, dry, dull skin. You are already taking supplements and eating foods that contain essential fatty acids. For best skin results, however, essential fatty acids should be applied directly to the skin. Gamma linoleic acid (GLA) is the primary essential fatty acid in the skin. Look for products that list essential fatty acids or gamma linoleic acid on the label. Today's high-tech moisturizers are not greasy and will be absorbed nicely by your skin. You can use the same moisturizer for morning and night, although some people prefer to use a heavier cream at night.

Some good-quality moisturizers and their sources are as follows:

- Gioni Protective Day Wear and Gioni Rejuvenative Night Cream developed by Dermatology Associates of San Diego County. For information call 1-800-450-0007.
- Insulation by Prescriptives. Available at department stores.
- Essential Moisture (with GLA) by Ecological Formulas: For information call 1-800-888-4585.

Now You See It . . .

As you implement my skin care regimen, I would like you to keep track of your progress by doing the "wrinkle test." Find one small wrinkle or one fine line on your face. Draw a simple sketch of your face, including that one wrinkle or line, so that you remember where it is. Put the picture away. After you have followed my skin care regimen for ten weeks, take out the picture and compare it to your face. The wrinkle should look noticeably better—that is, if you can still find it!

YOUR SKIN CARE REGIMEN

The Night Before: Getting Started

The Age Loss Program's skin care regimen is designed to accommodate the needs of busy people and should not take more than a few minutes a day to implement. I do recommend, however, that you begin the skin care regimen on a weekend or on a morning when you don't have to rush out of the house. In this way you can familiarize yourself with the basic routine.

The night before you begin the skin care regimen, you should prepare your skin by giving yourself a ten-minute herbal face sauna. This is not only a wonderful way to soften and deep-clean your skin, but most people find it a highly relaxing and enjoyable experience.

For your face sauna you will need a prepackaged mixture of dried herbs from your local herb shop (Body Shop or Aveda) or health food store. If you have time, you can create your own herbal mixture. My favorite mix is two tablespoons of lavender and one tablespoon each of orange blossoms, peppermint, chamomile, and fennel seeds.

THE HERBAL FACE SAUNA
Boil one quart of water. Mix in the herbs. Turn off the heat and cover the pot for two minutes. Remove the pot from the heat and put it on a table. Sit or stand about one foot away. Make a tentlike cover out of a towel and cover your head as you lean over the hot pot. Close your eyes and take a few deep, relaxing breaths. You may want to listen to soothing music. Steam your face. Wait ten minutes. Splash cool water on your face and apply your moisturizer. Your skin will be ultra-clean and radiate with good health, and tomorrow morning you will be ready to begin your skin care program.

Your Morning Regimen

1. Always start with a clean face and neck. Before you apply any skin product to your face or neck, make sure that your face is absolutely clean. Splash warm (not hot) water on your face and neck. Put a small amount of a mild, nonsoap cleanser in your hand and rub it into your face and neck. (Be sure to use as mild a cleanser as possible. Particularly gentle are soaps and cleansers that contain chamomile extract, such as CamoCare Chamomile Cleansing Therapy and Basis Soap for sensitive skin.) Rinse by splashing warm water on your face at least ten times. Lightly pat dry with a soft towel. Don't tug or pull at your face.

2. Apply vitamin C serum or cream. Gently rub a small amount of vitamin C cream or serum on your face and on the back, sides, and front of your neck. Vitamin C should always be the first cream to touch the skin so it can be absorbed immediately. If you want to use a vitamin C product under your eyes, be sure to use only weaker strength products designed for use in this sensitive area. Use just enough to cover the skin with a thin layer. Do not assume that if a little vitamin C is good, a lot is even better. *A little vitamin C goes a long way, and too much can be irritating.*

Whatever your skin type, vitamin C cream may sting slightly after you apply it, but any discomfort should disappear within a few seconds.

Note for men: Some men prefer to shave before applying vitamin C serum or cream, but since vitamin C may cause momentary stinging, you may want to shave after applying it if you have sensitive skin.

Wait 5 minutes to allow the vitamin C to be fully absorbed by your skin before shaving or applying other products.

3. Apply moisturizer. Now that you have applied your vitamin C cream, you are ready to use moisturizer. Splash some cool water on your face. Pat dry so that the skin is still slightly wet. Gently massage a fine layer of moisturizer into your face and neck.

4. Apply your sun protection. Sunscreen should be applied at least half an hour before going outdoors so it can be absorbed into your skin. Sunblock can be applied right before going outside since it is not absorbed into the skin.

Use at least half a teaspoon of sunscreen or sunblock for your face, neck, and hands. The biggest mistake that people make is that they do not use enough sun protection and are therefore not getting the full benefit. Gently massage the sunscreen or sunblock evenly into your skin. Be careful not to get it into your eyes because it can cause irritation.

Always reapply sunscreen or sunblock after swimming or engaging in vigorous activity that causes you to perspire.

Note for women: You are now ready to apply make-up and start your day. Be sure to bring the following items that you will need to reapply later: sun protection and moisturizer.

Your Midday Skin Care Regimen

1. Reapply your sun protection. Your sunscreen or sunblock can wear off over time. Reapply your sunscreen at lunchtime if you are going to be outdoors in the afternoon.

2. Reapply your moisturizer. This should be done if you have normal to dry skin. If you have oily skin, skip this step.

3. Spritz your face with water. Do this periodically to restore moisture.

Your Evening Skin Care Regimen

1. Always start out with a clean face and neck. If you wear makeup, be sure to remove all traces of it. If you use waterproof eye makeup, you will need a gentle eye makeup remover. Wash your face as you did in the morning.

2. Apply alpha hydroxy acid (AHA) cream or lotion. Always apply your AHA product to clean skin and wait about half an hour before putting on your retinol cream and moisturizer. This will give the AHA time to penetrate your skin and avoid diluting it.

If you have dry skin, use an AHA cream. If AHA makes your skin too dry, or if you find it irritating, use a low percentage AHA cream only every other day or even every second or third day.

Do not apply an AHA lotion or cream close to your eyes or on your eyelids because it can cause irritation and discomfort. If you have puffy or lined areas under your eyes, use only an AHA cream designed for that sensitive area.

3. Apply your retinol cream. Put a *small* dab of retinol cream in your hand and rub it gently on your face and neck. Do not apply retinol near your eyes. Let the retinol cream absorb into your skin for about ten minutes before applying moisturizer. People with sensitive skin may experience mild tingling or redness. If you find that retinol cream irritates your skin, try using it every other day instead of every day or on nights when you're not using AHA.

4. Reapply your moisturizer Spray cool water on your face. Pat dry but leave the skin slightly moist. Gently massage moisture cream into your skin.

Repeat the entire process every day for the next ten weeks.

If you are conscientious about following the Age Loss Program's skin care regimen, by the end of ten weeks you will see wonderful results. Your skin will be smoother, fresher, and more youthful-looking.

If you want to maintain your new skin, continue this

program. You will see such a marked improvement that, I guarantee, you will want to make this part of your daily regimen. The best thing you can do to prevent further sun damage is to stay out of the sun and wear your sunscreen or sunblock every day. You can, of course, continue your skin care regimen indefinitely, and this will help keep you looking ten years younger!

Step 4

⟋

REGAIN TEN YEARS OF MUSCLE

Develop a youthful, sleeker body
Restore lean body mass
Become stronger, slimmer, and sexier

BY FOLLOWING MY SUPPLEMENT and food plan, you will lose fat and gain muscle. Now I am going to show you another way to reclaim (and maintain) the muscle tone and strength that time has eroded. More important, I am going to show you how easy it is to feel good about your body again.

Step 4 describes my easy and painless exercise routine. Now I know what many of you are thinking: "Do I have to?" Frankly, if you follow the other steps that I recommend in this book, you will see results whether or not you follow my workout routine. But the effects of my supplement and food plan will be vastly enhanced if done in conjunction with this routine. Since you will also be doing yourself a lot of good, I urge you not to skip this step.

You will also see that an effective exercise routine doesn't have to be hard or time-consuming. The routine was designed with the assistance of Daren Gregson, Ph.D., the exercise physiologist at the Whitaker Wellness Center. Daren has worked with thousands of patients and understands what you want most in an exercise routine: You want it to be simple, yet you want fast results. Toward those goals we have created a very effective and efficient routine. By investing a minimal amount of time and effort you can reap enormous gains. It is also a progressive routine. You start slowly and, as you grow "younger" and more fit, you do more because you actually want to. By the end of ten weeks you will feel mentally and physically recharged, and healthier and happier than you have felt in years.

My Age Loss Program's workout routine does not restrict you to one activity. As you will see, you have a choice of five basic exercises: treadmill walking, outdoor walking, stationary cycling, outdoor cycling, and swimming. All of these exercises will burn fat and strengthen muscle tone in large muscle groups, especially in the lower body. You can choose one or several. You will never be stuck doing something that you don't like, nor will you get bored.

Finally, you don't have to be in great shape to start or benefit from my workout routine. In fact, it is ideal for the majority of folks who have not been on a regular exercise schedule and need to make up for lost time.

Inactivity Speeds Up Aging

I've said repeatedly that inaction accelerates aging. So does inactivity. To resist the forces of aging you need to do a minimum amount of exercise every week.

As we get older, the number and strength of our muscle fibers decrease. Starting as young as age thirty, we lose an average of two to four pounds of muscle a decade. In addition, many of us gain weight as we age, and muscle atrophy is concealed by those extra pounds of fat. Eventually, though, we notice a loss of flexibility as our atrophying muscles tighten and lose their range of motion. You may find that you can't get up from a chair as easily as you used to or that you can't bend over or crouch without feeling stiffness or pain. This is a sign that you need to rebuild your muscles.

Why do our muscles age? Several factors contribute to "muscle meltdown." It is partly a result of the energy drain that turns formerly active people into "couch potatoes" practically overnight. Men and women who used to find it possible—even refreshing—to run to the gym at the end of a hectic day suddenly find that all they want to do is go home, eat dinner, and "veg out" by the tube. (Clearly, these folks are not taking their "Energizers.")

Exercise not only strengthens muscles but stimulates the repair mechanism within the muscles so that new muscle is formed. If we don't exercise, even for a few weeks, our muscles will weaken significantly. In fact, if you stop exercising for just six weeks, you will lose about 50 percent of your muscle strength. (The good news here is that if you start exercising, you can quickly recover what you've lost.)

Muscle cells are particularly vulnerable to free radical attack. Free radicals injure cells and also make it difficult for muscle cells to repair themselves. As we lose our antioxidant balance, we lose the battle against free radicals, and muscle simply disappears. My Age Loss Program's supplement plan includes high doses of particular antioxidants that will restore your body's natural antioxidant defense system. This will prevent further muscle damage and stimulate the muscle cells to repair and heal themselves. But that is just the first step.

The way to prevent and to cure muscle loss is through exercise. Researchers have shown that if we exercise consistently, we can maintain much of our youthful musculature. In one groundbreaking study, researchers at the University of Colorado examined the body fat content of thirty female endurance athletes ranging in age from twenty-three to fifty-six. The researchers were surprised to find that regardless of age the women showed no significant difference in levels of body fat. In other words, the oldest women had the same sleek, lean bodies as the youngest women! This tells us that a decrease in muscle is not an inevitable part of aging. It tells us that if we stay physically active throughout our lives, we can maximize muscle tone and minimize fat.

This doesn't mean that you have to be an endurance athlete to maintain your muscles and enjoy the full benefits of exercise. The key is to maintain a consistent level of moderate exercise.

Age Loss Rule: It's Never Too Late!

The best thing you can do to maintain muscle mass is to *use* your muscles, and it's never too late to start. It doesn't matter whether you are thirty-nine or ninety-nine. Nor does it matter that you haven't exercised in years. What is truly remarkable about even moderate exercise is that, like the Age Loss Program itself, it can benefit us all. It does so in the following ways:

1. Exercise restores youthful metabolism. Muscle is the "engine" that burns calories. In adults, about one-third of energy expenditure is due to muscular activity. The bigger and stronger our muscles, the more calories we burn. Conversely, as muscle shrinks, the fewer calories we burn. Our metabolism slows, and those unburned calories are stored as fat. We develop "middle-age spread." As we rebuild muscle, we are also making our metabolism younger.

2. Exercise rejuvenates the heart. When I talk about muscle, I'm not just talking about biceps and triceps. Don't forget that the heart is also a muscle and that exercise is essential for the health of this vital organ. Indeed, regular exercise reduces the risk of developing heart disease by as much as half.

3. Exercise strengthens bones. About one-third of all women and 15 percent of all men will suffer from osteoporosis, the thinning of bone that makes them vulnerable to fractures. Weight-bearing exercise (such as walking, running, and jogging) can help maintain bone mass.

4. Exercise makes you feel good. Ever notice how exercise puts you in a better mood? It's not just your imagination. Exercise stimulates your brain to produce hormones called endorphins, natural painkillers and mood enhancers. That is why exercise produces such a wonderful "natural high."

Now that you know all the great benefits of exercise, I hope you are ready to begin the workout. One note of caution: If you are over forty, or have a history of a medical problem, call your physician before beginning this or any other exercise program. Chances are that your doctor will be delighted you want to exercise, but in some cases he or she may may want you to take a simple exercise stress test to check your heart function.

GET READY . . .

As noted earlier, my Age Loss Program's workout routine lets you choose from five different activities: treadmill walking, outdoor walking, stationary cycling, outdoor cycling, and swimming. You can pick one of these activities or mix them up. It doesn't matter as long as you exercise at least three times a week.

Obviously, I want you to select the activities that you will enjoy best. Also keep in mind these other considerations:

- EQUIPMENT
  Do you have access to the right equipment? Walking outdoors is the only activity on the list that does not require

special equipment other than a comfortable pair of shoes. Many of you may already have stationary bikes or treadmills that are probably gathering dust. Now is a good time to dust them off and put them to good use. If you don't own your own equipment, check out the facilities at a local health club, gym, or Y. I'm willing to bet that many of you are already paid members of a health club even though you haven't been there in weeks or months. If so, get back in there. If not, try to find one that offers a trial membership for a small fee.

- **WEATHER**

  Many people, myself included, prefer outdoor exercise. I find that there is nothing more invigorating than a brisk walk or bicycle ride on a bright, sunny day. Luckily, I live in southern California where the weather is usually good. If you live in a less hospitable climate, choose an exercise that you can do indoors on days that are too hot, cold, or wet.

- **PHYSICAL CONDITION**

  Do you have any physical limitations? Not every exercise is for everyone or every body. For example, if you have chronic knee or heel problems, walking may aggravate your condition, and therefore working out on a stationary bike may be your best bet. Stationary bikes protect your bones and joints from undue stress while improving muscle tone, burning fat, and giving you a good cardiovascular workout. If you have any orthopedic injuries, ask your doctor which exercise is best for you.

Each particular exercise in the workout routine has its advantages and disadvantages. Here are some things you need to know before devising your routine.

Treadmill Walking

The advantage of treadmill walking is that it is done indoors and therefore you can exercise in any kind of weather. You may find outdoor walking boring, but when you are on a treadmill, you can read a magazine or even watch television to pass the time.

The disadvantage is that you either have to own a treadmill or have access to one at your local gym or health club. Since treadmills are incredibly popular, you will find that most gyms and health clubs have at least one—if not several. The downside is that you may have to wait to use a treadmill if you tend to go to the gym or health club at peak hours when it is crowded. And if you are trying to fit your workout in during your lunch hour or before work, this may get aggravating—which defeats the whole purpose of exercise! If you decide to join a gym, check out how many treadmills are available and when the busiest times are so that you can avoid "rush hours."

There is another advantage to treadmill walking that you should take into consideration. As I will explain later, during your workout routine, you will be monitoring your heart rate. You can program your training heart rate on a computerized treadmill, which will make it easy for you to control the intensity of your workout. (If you don't use a treadmill, don't worry. This is still relatively easy to do, as will be explained on page 146.)

Treadmill walking is easy, but it does require some balance and coordination. If you tend to lose your balance easily, I do not recommend using a treadmill. The only downside to using a treadmill (and outdoor walking) is that it can be stressful on your heels and feet. If you have heel pain or foot pain, use a stationary bicycle instead. Otherwise, treadmill walking is a safe, convenient way to get the job done.

Outdoor Walking

Outdoor walking is a wonderful way to exercise. It requires no special equipment other than a good pair of walking shoes and a pedometer to measure your speed. It is easy and free, and being outdoors on a great day can send your spirits soaring.

Walking outdoors on a bad day, however, can be downright depressing, and only the most committed walkers are motivated enough to do it. If you have access to an indoor track, plan to move indoors in inclement weather. If you don't, perhaps you will want to use a treadmill on nasty days and walk outside on nice days. Whatever you do, don't let the weather come between you and your workout.

If you walk outdoors, do not walk in isolated areas by yourself and try to vary your route so that you don't get bored with the scenery. You can listen to music through headphones if you like, but be sure that you can still hear traffic noise. If possible, try to find someone who will walk with you. It is a relaxing way to keep up with friends, and it makes the time go faster.

Stationary Cycling

There are many advantages to stationary cycling and only one big disadvantage. As noted earlier, it is not a weight-bearing exercise and has minimum benefits for maintaining bone strength. Therefore, it is not the best choice if you are worried about osteoporosis.

Because it is not a weight-bearing exercise, stationary cycling is recommended for people with knee or foot problems. It spares the joints the kind of wear and tear that can cause arthritic flare-ups. Also, since it is done indoors at home or at the gym or health club, you don't have to worry about bad weather breaking your routine. You also don't have to worry about traffic as you do if you cycle on the roads.

Similar to treadmill walking, on most stationary cycles you can program in your training heart rate, which makes it easy to control the intensity of your workout. You can also read or watch television while you are cycling, which makes the time go faster.

Outdoor Cycling

Having spent ten weeks pedaling cross-country, I can tell you that there is nothing quite as exhilarating as listening to the whistle of the wind as you take in the scenery. Cycling is a wonderful way to spend some meaningful time with yourself.

Cycling can be hectic, however, if you must dart in and out of traffic and your lungs fill with gasoline fumes. If you do not live in an area conducive to outdoor cycling, don't do it.

Outdoor cycling is particularly good exercise for people with arthritic knees as long as the seat is set at the right height so that the knees are not hyperextended or bent more than 90 degrees.

Never go cycling without a helmet; it is dangerous. A helmet prevents the most serious head injuries caused by falls. You should also wear tinted shatterproof goggles or sunglasses to protect your eyes from dust, stones, and other pieces of flying debris. I also recommend that you attach a speedometer to your bicycle if you don't already have one to track your progress.

Swimming

Swimming is a particularly good choice for people who suffer from arthritis and/or are overweight. The buoyancy of the water reduces stress on joints and bones, sparing them undue stress. At the same time, swimming at a brisk pace gives you a great cardiovascular workout and strengthens and improves nearly all muscle groups.

Swimming is not for everyone. Some people may find that their skin or eyes are irritated by chlorine or that it dries out their hair. Wearing goggles and showering immediately after swimming can usually solve these problems. People who are prone to inner ear infections may also want to avoid swimming since infection of the ear canal is a fairly common problem among swimmers.

On the upside, swimming can be a refreshing and exhilarating way to burn those calories and build muscle.

Getting Motivated

Once you select your exercise routine, you need to give some serious thought to how you are going to incorporate it into your life. I have found it is helpful to do the following:

1. Establish a set time for exercise. If you do not schedule it into your week as you would any other important business date or function, you will too easily put it off. To be safe, schedule forty-five minutes three days a week for the next ten weeks. This is a gradual program, and during weeks one and two, your workout should take only half an hour. By the end of ten weeks you will be in such good shape that you will be able to work out longer. Also, don't forget to allow time for showering, and so forth, if you are on a tight schedule.

For most people the best times to exercise are either early in the morning before work, during lunch hour, or early evening after work. It is better to exercise every other day rather than every day. The day off will give your muscles time to rest and repair. Don't schedule exercise too late in the evening; if you do, you may find it difficult to fall asleep. Ideally, you should allow yourself at least two to three hours of downtime before going to sleep to avoid a restless night.

2. Make it social. Try to schedule your workout with a spouse or a friend. That way you will be less likely to skip your exercise routine because someone else is counting on you. Several years ago I had a standing date to jog at six o'clock every morning with two of my neighbors. I know that had I not felt duty bound to exercise with my partners, I would have stayed in bed many mornings.

3. Make it meaningful. Many worthwhile charities sponsor walks, runs, and bike rides to raise money for their cause. Use the ten weeks you are on the Age Loss Program's exercise routine as an opportunity to train for such an event. Check with your favorite charities to see what events are coming up. It is a wonderful way to do something for yourself and others.

THE BASICS

The Age Loss Program's exercise routine is designed to reinvigorate your body quickly and efficiently. It is a training program in which each session is divided into two different segments or intervals. During each interval you will begin at a slow, easy pace (for two to three minutes), work up to a harder pace (for eight to fifteen minutes), and then end at a slow, easy pace (for two to three minutes). You will then repeat the segment. Do not stop in between intervals. The big advantage of interval training is that you can progress more rapidly than if you followed a traditional training program because you alternate between bursts of intense activity (which builds up endurance faster) and a more relaxed pace in which your body can rest. In other words, by following this routine you can achieve more in a shorter period of time. The only time you will not be doing interval training is during weeks one and two when you will work out in one continuous twenty-minute session in order to ease your body into the routine.

The workout is designed to enhance your cardiovascular health, improve your muscle strength and tone, and improve your appearance. The ten-week workout routine progresses in stages. Every two weeks, as you become more fit, you will advance to a more challenging level and work out a longer period of time.

Always Warm Up

Before you do any type of exercise, spend at least five minutes warming up your muscles. Whether you march or jog in place at a very easy pace, walk on your treadmill, pedal on your bike at an easy pace, or swim a few casual laps, the purpose of the warm-up is to increase the blood flow to the muscles, which will allow them to relax and contract more smoothly. If you do not warm up properly before you exercise, particularly if you have not been exercising regularly, you risk injuring a muscle. Your warm-up exercise should be done at an easy pace. When you break a light sweat, it is a sign that you are properly warmed up.

Don't Forget to Stretch

After your warm-up, take five minutes to stretch out the muscles in your legs, arms, and back. Stretching enhances flexibility and prepares your muscles for physical activity. It also makes you feel good. Here is one of the best ways to stretch: Sit on the floor with your legs extended, straight in front of you. Bend from the waist to try to touch your toes with your fingertips. Do not lock your knees and don't be overzealous. Never force a stretch or bounce into it. Simply stretch out your arms as far as you can without causing pain and then hold the stretch for about ten seconds. Repeat the exercise ten times.

To stretch your hamstrings (the muscles behind your

thigh), sit on the edge of your bed with one foot on the floor and the other leg extended and slightly bent. Bend from the waist and slowly reach toward the toes of the extended leg. Hold the stretch for about fifteen seconds, then sit up. Again, don't force it. Simply stretch as far as you can and hold it for ten seconds. Repeat the exercise ten times and then switch legs.

Establish Your Training Heart Rate

When you exercise, your heart will obviously beat faster than when you are at rest. Although it is good to exercise your heart muscle, you don't want to overdo it. You therefore need to establish a *training heart rate* in which you can exercise safely, comfortably, and effectively. To figure out your training heart rate, you will need to know your *high* training heart rate and your *low* training heart rate. When you exercise, you generally want your heart rate to fall within these two numbers.

Use this simple formula, which is based on your age, to figure out your training heart rates. The math is not hard, but it's a lot easier if you use a calculator. If you write down all your answers, you will have to do this only once.

1. Determine your *maximum* heart rate. The maximum heart rate helps determine training heart rate. To find this number, subtract your age from 220. Example: If you are 50 years old: 220 less 50 = 170 beats per minute.
2. Determine your *low* training heart rate. To do this, multiply your high heart rate by .65. Example: 170 x .65 = 110 beats per minute.
3. Determine your *high* training heart rate. To do this, multiply your maximum heart rate by .75. Example: 170 x .75 = 127 beats per minute.

Use your low training heart rate and high training heart rate as a guide. If you work below your low training heart rate, you are not getting enough of a workout, and if you work above your high training heart rate, you may be overdoing it. There is one exception to this rule. For the first two weeks of the Age Loss Program, I want you to take it very easy and purposefully work *below* your low training heart rate. Specifically, I want you to work at 85 percent of your low training heart rate. To determine this, multiply your low training heart rate by .85. Example: 110 x .85 = 93 beats per minute.

For the following eight weeks I will tell you to aim at either your low training heart rate or high training heart rate. If you are below your high training heart rate, you can work a bit harder. If you are above it, slow down. As the weeks progress, your exercise will move you to a gradually higher rate until you reach your high training heart rate.

How Do I Measure My Training Heart Rate?

In order to keep track of your heart rate, you need to know how to take your pulse. The easiest way to do this is to place two fingers at the side of your neck, next to your carotid artery. You will feel the pulsing of your blood through the artery. Measure the number of beats or pulses you feel in ten seconds. To determine your heartbeat per minute, multiply that number by six. For example, if you count 20 beats in ten seconds, you multiply that number by six (to make a full minute). This equals 120. That means your heart is working at a rate of 120 beats per minute.

When you begin your workout, you will gradually pick up speed until you reach your goal. For example, on Week One if you're using a treadmill, you will slowly increase the intensity of your workout until you reach three miles per hour, the goal for that week. At the end of the twenty-minute workout (before you cool), take your pulse to measure your training heart rate. If your training heart rate is where it should be, then continue to exercise at that level. If your training heart rate is too low, pick up your pace until you achieve the right training heart rate.

On the weeks that you do interval training, you will check your training heart rate immediately following the first workout segment, and you will adjust your pace accordingly.

Note to swimmers: If you choose swimming as your activity, due to the horizontal position of your body your training heart rate will be about ten points lower than if you choose one of the other activities. So if your low training heart rate is normally 110, on the days that you swim it will be 100.

Always Cool Down

After you have completed your workout, slowly wind down your exercise before stopping completely. This gives your heart and muscles a chance to return to normal, and it can prevent a sudden drop in blood pressure that can make you feel faint.

Replenish Lost Fluid and Nutrients

Be sure to drink one to two glasses of water after you exercise to replace lost fluids. For best results eat a light meal and take your supplements immediately following exercise. You need to replenish the nutrients you used up during the workout. This is also the time that your body is most likely to burn calories and less likely to store them as fat.

... Go!

Get moving! You are now ready to begin the Age Loss Program's workout routine.

Weeks One and Two

Before you begin, don't forget to do your five-minute warm-up and stretching exercises.

As you may recall, you will not be doing an interval program for Weeks One and Two. Instead, you will do your chosen activity for a *continuous* twenty minutes. Select from any of the activities listed below. Start out at a slow pace and work up to the designated pace. At the end of twenty minutes you will take your pulse to check your training heart rate. If it is too high, reduce your pace during your next exercise session. If it is too low, pick up your pace a bit. Slow down for two to three minutes before discontinuing your activity. Some of you may be in better shape than others, and the exercise segment that I've provided for Weeks One and Two may not be rigorous enough for you. If that is the case, simply start out with Weeks Three and Four.

Don't forget to check your training heart rate after you have completed your twenty-minute workout. You should aim to work at .85 percent of your low training heart rate.

Activity	Designated Goal
Treadmill walking	Walk at a pace of 3 mph
Outdoor walking	Walk at a pace of 3 mph (20 minutes for each mile)
Stationary cycling	Set resistance at 70 rpm
Outdoor cycling	Ride at a rate of 9 mph ($6^1/_2$ minutes for each mile)
Swimming	Swim at a speed of 2.5 minutes per lap (1 lap = 1 length of the pool or 50 yards)

Weeks Three and Four

Before you begin, don't forget to do your five-minute warm-up and stretching exercises.

After you have completed two weeks of exercise, I'm sure that you will already feel different. In fact, you should be able to pick up the pace a bit without much additional effort—and that's exactly what I suggest you do for Weeks Three and Four. Now you are ready to begin the interval training part of this routine, which will include two short segments. During each segment you will work at a very easy pace for three minutes, pick up your speed to reach the designated goal for eight minutes, and then return to a very easy pace for three minutes. Each time you exercise, you will do two complete segments. When you are working the hardest, during the eight-minute stint, aim for your *low* training heart rate. You will take your pulse to check your training heart rate only once—after you have completed the first eight minutes at your designated goal. If it is too fast or too slow, adjust your workout accordingly for the second segment. Choose from any of the activities listed below.

Activity	Designated Goal for 8 Minutes
Treadmill walking	Walk at a pace of 3.5 mph
Outdoor walking	Walk at a pace of 3.5 mph (17 minutes for each mile)
Stationary cycling	Set resistance equal to low training heart rate. (If you cannot program this information into your bike, you will have to experiment a bit by trying a few different levels of resistance and then checking your pulse.)

Outdoor cycling	Ride at a rate of 10 mph (6 minutes for each mile)
Swimming	Swim at a speed of 2.5 minutes per lap (1 lap = 1 length of the pool or 50 yards)

Weeks Five and Six

Before you begin, don't forget to do your five-minute warm-up and stretching exercises.

Take a deep breath. You are almost halfway there. You should be noticing a marked improvement in how you look and feel. Do you have more energy? Have you lost weight and firmed up? For the next two weeks I am going to push you a bit more so that you work at your *high* training heart rate. By now you are probably in such great shape, this will be a snap!

This time, during each segment, you will work at a very easy pace for three minutes, pick up your speed and work at your high training heart rate for ten minutes, and then return to a very easy pace for three minutes. You will take your pulse to check your training heart rate only once, after completing the first ten minutes at your designated goal. If your training heart rate is high or too low, adjust your workout accordingly for the second segment. Choose from any of the activities listed below.

Activity	**Designated Goal for 10 Minutes**
Treadmill walking	Walk at a pace of 4 mph
Outdoor walking	Walk at a pace of 4 mph (15 minutes for each mile)
Stationary cycling	Set resistance equal to high training heart rate
Outdoor cycling	Ride at a rate of 10.5 mph (5$^1/_2$ minutes for each mile)

151

| Swimming | Swim at a speed of 2 minutes per lap (1 lap = 1 length of the pool or 50 yards) |

Weeks Seven and Eight

Before you begin, don't forget to do your five-minute warm-up and stretching exercises.

As you will see, by Weeks Seven and Eight, you should note a vast improvement in your body and endurance rate. Keep up the good work!

This time during each segment you will work at a very easy pace for two minutes, pick up your speed to reach the designated goal for twelve minutes, and then return to a very easy pace for two minutes. During the twelve-minute stint, when you are working the hardest, aim for your *high* training heart rate. You will take your pulse to check your training heart rate only once, after completing the first twelve minutes at your designated goal. If it is too high or too low, adjust your workout accordingly for the second segment. Choose from any of the activities listed below.

Activity	Designated Goal for 12 Minutes
Treadmill walking	Walk at a pace of 4.5 mph
Outdoor walking	Walk at a pace of 4.5 mph (13 minutes for each mile)
Stationary cycling	Set resistance equal to high training heart rate
Outdoor cycling	Ride at a rate of 12 mph (5 minutes for each mile)
Swimming	Swim at a speed of 1.5 minutes per lap (1 lap = 1 length of the pool or 50 yards)

152

Weeks Nine and Ten

Before you begin, don't forget to do your five-minute warm-up and stretching exercises.

The goal that I have set for the last two weeks of your workout is more demanding, but by now you should be in such good shape that you are ready for the challenge.

This time during each segment you will work at a very easy pace for two minutes, pick up your speed to reach the designated goal for fifteen minutes, and then return to a very easy pace for two minutes. During the fifteen-minute stint, when you are working your hardest, aim for your *high* training heart rate. Take your pulse to check your training heart rate only once, after completing the first fifteen minutes at your designated goal. If it is too high or too low, adjust your workout accordingly for the second segment. Choose from any of the activities listed below.

Activity	Designated Goal for 15 Minutes
Treadmill walking	Walk at a pace of 5 mph
Outdoor walking	Walk at a pace of 5 mph (12 minutes for each mile)
Stationary cycling	Set resistance equal to high training heart rate
Outdoor cycling	Ride at a rate of 13 mph ($4^1/_2$ minutes for each mile)
Swimming	Swim at a speed of 1.5 minutes per lap (1 lap = 1 length of the pool or 50 yards)

WHAT IF I FEEL. . . .

When you begin a new exercise program, you are liable to experience sensations that you haven't felt before, and you may not be able to distinguish normal aches and pains from the more serious ones. If you have any unusual symptoms during exercise—for example, if you feel dizzy or weak or have any pain—stop your activity and consult a doctor immediately. But sometimes symptoms aren't so obvious. Here are some answers to questions that I am commonly asked about exercise:

What if my heart starts to pound while I am exercising?

Your heart is going to beat faster during vigorous exercise, and it may even feel as though it is pounding. This symptom by itself should not cause alarm. If your heartbeat is very irregular, however, and feels as if it is fluttering or jumping in your chest, or there is a sudden rapid burst of heartbeats, you should stop exercising and contact your doctor. It may be nothing, but it could also be a sign of a cardiac rhythm disorder, which may require attention.

What if I have difficulty catching my breath after I stop exercising?

It's normal to be breathless for a few minutes after a vigorous workout, but if it lasts for more than ten minutes, it is a sign that you are overtaxing your heart and lungs. Slow down! Stay at the low training heart rate. As a general rule, make sure that while you are exercising, you are not too out of breath to be understood by a companion.

What if I sweat a lot?

Sweating is a normal reaction when your body is overheated. It is nothing to worry about. But breaking into a cold sweat is a different story, especially if it is accompanied by a sudden loss of coordination or confusion. If this happens to you, stop exercising and lie down with your feet elevated. Check with your doctor before resuming your exercise routine.

What if I get a stitch in my side?

A side stitch (a pain under the ribs while exercising) is caused by a spasm of the diaphragm muscle. If this happens while you are exercising, gradually reduce your speed and then sit down in a chair or on the ground. Lean forward so that you push your abdomen against your diaphragm. This should help relieve the spasm.

What if I feel nausea or vomit immediately following exercise?

This is a sign that you are not getting enough oxygen to your intestines. You are either exercising too vigorously or not taking enough time to cool down. Cut back on your exercise and take more time cooling down.

What if my muscles feel sore the day after I exercise?

It is normal to feel some muscle ache after exercise; however, if you are in a great deal of discomfort, it could be a sign that you are not cooling down enough after your workout. Never discontinue exercise abruptly. Slowly wind down so that your muscles can relax gradually, which will help prevent muscle pain the next day.

What if I feel exhausted the day after I exercise?

You may be exercising at too vigorous a level. Stay at the low training heart rate or even below. Once you build endurance, you can gradually increase your exercise level.

Congratulations. You have completed your ten-week workout and should feel and see dramatic changes in both your body and your mind. You should feel more energetic and alert than you have felt in a long time. If you want to continue to feel vigorous and strong, make exercise a regular part of your life.

Step 5

∅

BOOST YOUR BRAIN POWER

Sharpen your thinking

Improve your powers of concentration

Regain your mental edge

I do my brain exercises and take my brain boosters every day, and now I'm sharper than ever. I can mentally spar with the twenty-five-year-old "kids" at the office. They have trouble keeping up with me.

JACK M., 55

Since I began Dr. Whitaker's program, the biggest change I've noticed is that my memory has improved dramatically. Before I started the program, I just didn't have the power of concentration that I used to. Now my brain is functioning beautifully. My memory is back. I can remember phone numbers. I can remember that I have an appointment without looking at my date book. I've recouped so much—it's like the way I used to be.

LARRY P., 69

Do you have trouble remembering names? Do you find yourself constantly searching for your car keys or your wallet? Is it just a little more difficult for you to concentrate than it used to be? If you answered yes to any of these questions, you're not alone. In fact, you're in good company. These are the kinds of subtle mental changes that typically begin during midlife. They are not serious or unusual. Nor are they irreversible. If you follow the Age Loss Program to boost your brain power, you can regain much of what you have lost and will be as smart and sharp as you were before!

Of all the problems that people associate with growing older, there is none more disconcerting than the sensation that we are "losing it" mentally. Let me tell you about a patient of mine, Susan, fifty-two, who found these mental changes quite disturbing. Susan is an accountant who prides herself on her ability to remember dates, names, and other details that are relevant to her clients. When Susan became menopausal, however, she began to notice a marked change in her ability to recall information. She had difficulty concentrating and was easily distracted. When she came to see me, she was in the midst of a frenetic "tax season." Practically in tears, Susan said that she was on a downward spiral that she feared would lead to the inability to perform her job.

Susan was greatly relieved to know that I have heard similar complaints from literally thousands of men and women her age, and that everything she was experiencing was normal. A name or phone number forgotten, difficulty coming up with the right words, or finding that you don't have the mental stamina you once had is not an uncommon occurrence for people in their middle years and older. It is such a common occurrence that the National Institute of Mental Health has even given it a name: Age Associated Memory Impairment. Some people may experience more memory or concentration problems than others, but very rarely do these changes signify that anything is seriously wrong.

To say that Susan's condition was common is not to say that it should not be remedied. Treating Susan's problem was reasonably simple. I was able to devise a program of brain boosting nutrition and supplements, stress reduction, and natural hormones that greatly reduced Susan's symptoms, and she is now performing her job better than ever.

It is important to understand that some very real changes in brain function can interfere with our ability to perform our jobs, pursue our interests, or even engage in social activity comfortably. The best news is that you can preserve and even enhance your memory and other aspects of mental function. Concentration, alertness, and ability to focus can also be strengthened, leading to improvements in problem-solving ability, productivity, and even IQ.

Your brain is vulnerable to the same destructive forces that accelerate aging throughout your body. All the steps of the Age Loss Program will have a beneficial effect on brain function, but there are some specific exercises you can do to maintain your mental edge and keep it razor sharp. Let me tell you a little about your brain and how it works.

WHAT MAKES YOUR BRAIN TICK

The human brain is the most complex, specialized, and mysterious organ in the body. It is also one of the most hard working. The brain coordinates all of the body's nervous activity, processes incoming sensory impulses, and is the repository of reasoning, intellect, memory, consciousness, and emotions.

Your brain requires constant nourishment to fuel its many activities. This constant supply of blood and oxygen is vital: Within minutes of nutrient deprivation, brain cells begin to die. If the supply of oxygen and nutrients is cut off, as in the case of a cerebral stroke, the brain will sustain injury.

The worker cells of the brain are called neurons, and they never rest. Neurons are in constant communication with one another via a vast network of tiny branchlike cells called dendrites that send and receive messages. We produce dendrites at a brisk pace when we are young, but as we get older, it becomes more difficult to make new dendrites. This is one of the reasons that we experience memory lapses and have difficulty learning new things.

The cells of the brain "talk" to one another by releasing chemicals called neurotransmitters. As we age, we also experience a decline in neurotransmitters by as much as 70 percent, which may also be a factor in brain aging.

Several hormones also influence overall brain functioning. Researchers have recently found that estrogen, testosterone, and DHEA, the hormones that regulate reproductive activity, are also neurotransmitters and play a major role in maintaining mood and mental function. The decline in these hormones is in part responsible for some of the age-related changes that occur in brain function.

It may surprise you to learn that your brain runs on electricity. I'm not joking. An electrical impulse is what prompts the "spilling" of neurotransmitters that enables nerve cells to carry on a conversation. We measure electrical activity with a test called an electroencephalogram (EEG). Electrical activity in the brain changes as we age, and there are distinct differences in the EEG of an older and younger person.

As you can see, your brain is a hotbed of activity, and to keep it functioning well, we need to replenish what time has taken away. There are several ways to boost brain power in just ten weeks. If you are following my Age Loss Program, you are already on the right track, but here are some additional things you can incorporate into your daily regimen—at least for the next ten weeks.

Boost Your Antioxidant Levels to Boost Brain Power

Do you ever use the expression "I'm getting rusty" to describe your inability to perform a task as well as you used to? Actually, it's a wonderful description of what happens to brains as we age.

Rust is caused by oxidative damage due to free radicals. Your brain is also vulnerable to damage by free radicals due to its extraordinary activity level. As mentioned earlier, the brain needs a continuous supply of blood and oxygen to produce enough energy to fuel this activity. The downside is that the more energy we produce, the more free radicals we produce. Also, brain cells are composed of more than 50 percent fat, and fat is especially prone to free radical damage.

If you want to preserve your brain function and prevent it from "rusting," you must get enough antioxidants from your food and supplements. The Age Loss Program's cuisine and supplement plan contains high amounts of protective antioxidants, including vitamins A, C, and E, beta-carotene, lipoic acid, and selenium, but perhaps the most effective supplement for the brain is ginkgo biloba, which you are already taking as a daily supplement.

GET SMART; GET GINKGO.
The herb ginkgo biloba contains special compounds called flavonoids, potent antioxidants that keep free radicals in check. The overall effect of ginkgo biloba supplementation is improved circulation and delivery of oxygen and nutrients, and nowhere is this more important than in the brain. (It also improves sexual performance, which is discussed in Step 6.)

Ginkgo biloba has been studied as a treatment for inadequate blood flow to the brain, and the results are extremely promising. A recent French study involved a group of sixty- to eighty-year-olds who had slight problems with mental function, the kind most of us experience. Volunteers were given ginkgo biloba supplements or a placebo. One hour later they took a battery of tests to determine their speed of information processing. The results of this test were astounding. After treatment with ginkgo biloba, the patients' scores improved so dramatically that they were close to the scores of young, healthy people! This study shows that ginkgo biloba can significantly benefit memory, even in individuals who have already demonstrated some memory loss. (The Age Loss ODA for ginkgo biloba is 120 milligrams daily.)

Control Stress Before It Controls You

Another agent of premature aging of the brain is chronic stress. Like the "fight or flight" reaction we have to perceived danger, there is a well-defined physiological response to chronic physical and emotional stress, and it begins with the release of stress hormones. These hormones quickly flood your tissues, including your brain, and initiate a cascade of physiological changes, putting you into a hyper-alert, energized state, ready to take on impending danger. A little excitement, an occasional rush of fear, irritation, or dread, is something that your body can handle. But chronic feelings of anxiety, fear, or anger, and even irritability, lack of control, overwork, lack of sleep, and the like, take their toll. High levels of these hormones are released and rarely have a chance to clear from your system. And as a general rule, the older we get, the longer they stay elevated.

Stress hormones have a decidedly negative effect on your brain. In animal studies, prolonged stress has been shown to accelerate brain aging and damage areas of the brain involved in learning and memory. Humans do not fare any better. In fact, researchers at McGill University in Montreal monitored the concentration of the blood levels of stress hormones in

130 healthy volunteers, age fifty-five to eighty-seven, over a five-year period. The researchers discovered that high blood levels of stress hormones correlate with subtle memory and attention problems. High levels of stress hormones have even been suggested as a possible cause of Alzheimer's disease.

Stress is part of our fast-paced society, and it's unavoidable. I know from my own experience, however, that chronic stress—deadlines, tight scheduling, and overcommitment—is a big factor in forgetfulness, lack of focus, and inability to concentrate. Taking control of your time and cutting back on a few things may be among the most important things you can do to improve cognitive function. Refer to Step 8 for some specific information on how to cope with stress.

Avoid Brain Poisons

Over the next ten weeks I want you to become aware of the drugs and medications that you put into your body. Many commonly prescribed drugs are literally brain poisons. Recreational drugs such as cocaine and amphetamines are extremely dangerous and can have very damaging effects on brain chemistry. But did you know that psychotropic drugs such as antidepressants, tranquilizers and even sleeping pills, can affect memory and alertness? Even common drugs, such as beta-blockers for high blood pressure, pain killers, antihistamines, diet pills, and glaucoma medications also interfere with brain function. Take a hard look at your medication list and work with your doctor to see what drugs you can eliminate in the interest of preserving your brain function.

Exercise Your Brain

As mentioned earlier, brain cells communicate with one another via tiny branchlike cells called dendrites. As we age, our ability to form dendrites declines, which is why our memory wanes and we have more difficulty learning new tasks. Dendrite growth peaks before adolescence. This is one of the reasons that children pick up languages, musical instruments, and other skills so readily while we adults struggle with them. If your child or grandchild has ever tried to teach you how to play a video game, you know what I'm talking about. Children's brains make connections faster. After puberty, the formation of new dendrites slows down, and at that point connections that are used frequently become permanent while those that are underutilized are lost. Through the years there is a constant "brain drain," resulting in fewer and fewer new dendrites.

When I was in medical school, we were taught that the adult brain was fully formed and that it could not grow new cells. Now we know better. We have learned that the brain is extremely resilient, even in adulthood, and that it has an amazing capacity to restore itself if it is given the proper stimulation. We have learned that if we use our brain by challenging ourselves mentally, we can build new nerve connections and strengthen neuron pathways. The result is increased brain power and a more youthful functioning brain.

Numerous studies on animals have demonstrated that intellectual challenges encourage neurons to branch out and create new connections, and there is compelling evidence that the same is true for humans.

In a fascinating study, Dr. David Snowden at the University of Kentucky, is monitoring a group of nuns living in a convent in Mankato, Minnesota. These nuns are remarkable not only because they live considerably longer than the general population but they also suffer significantly less dementia and Alzheimer's disease, even in their older years. They live healthy lives and have a strong social support structure, but beyond that, they have something which is even more important: an ethic of intellectual stimulation. They make it a point to read, play word games, do puzzles, work on their vocabularies, and continue to contribute to the convent in meaningful ways throughout their lives. Even more fascinating, brain scans show that the better educated nuns—those who teach, study, and continue to learn—have significantly more cortex, the area of the brain associated with language and reasoning, and more dendrites than the nuns whose work is less mentally stimulating, such as cooking and cleaning.

The exercise analogy is inevitable: Use it or lose it. Yes, optimal nutrition is vital, but even if you eat the best of diets and have a broad-spectrum nutritional supplement program, your cardiovascular and muscular fitness will suffer without exercise. The same is true of your brain and cognitive fitness.

Fun Drug-Free Ways to Improve Memory and Boost Your Brain Power

For the next ten weeks, try to live by these simple rules, and I guarantee that you will feel sharper and more mentally alert than you have in a long time.

- **Pump those neurons!** Exercise your brain daily to keep it fit. People who use their brains and who challenge themselves intellectually build extra neural connections. It is important to keep your brain working by absorbing new information each day.
- **Challenge your mind.** In order for these brain exercises to be effective, you must do different exercises on different days. The more you use your brain to perform a certain skill, the easier it becomes and the less likely that new dendrites will be formed. It is essential, therefore, to try a variety of challenging mental tasks and, most important, some new things that you have never done before.

- **Schedule specific times to exercise your brain.** To achieve the maximum benefit, you must approach these "brain workouts" in a systematic manner. For the next ten weeks schedule specific times in your day to do your brain exercises.
- **Turn off the TV!** For the ten weeks you are on the Age Loss Program, I urge you to watch as little television as possible. Watching television is the kind of passive activity that keeps your brain stagnant and it does not grow new cells. Devote the time that you would normally watch TV to performing your brain exercises.

It is essential that your brain exercises be enjoyable and a form of recreation, but to be effective they must also be challenging.

Here are some brain exercises that I like to do myself.

LISTEN TO MOZART.

Here's an easy one to get you started. One of the most enjoyable activities of life—listening to classical music—can actually boost your IQ. Researchers have dubbed this phenomenon "the Mozart effect." A 1993 study at the University of California in Irvine demonstrated that after listening to Mozart's "Sonata for Two Pianos in D Major, K448," thirty-six student volunteers temporarily increased their IQs by an average of nine points. Their average IQ was 110 without the benefit of music, but after listening to this music, their average IQ was 119. So far, Mozart is the only composer whose work has been shown to raise IQ levels. One of the investigators of this study, physicist Gordon Shaw, Ph.D., theorizes that the complex organization, themes, and rhythms of Mozart's music "open up" the electrical pathways in the brain that are involved in cognitive thinking and problem solving. What a delightful way to improve your mental functioning!

165

READ THE CLASSICS.

One of the most effective ways to stay sharp is to read. Among my patients I can always spot the avid readers. They are the ones who appear to be the most alert and ask the best questions. Choose something that suits your own tastes, but make it challenging. I've recently returned to the classics. You'll find that Charles Dickens's *A Tale of Two Cities* is a completely different book from the time that you read it in high school. Listening to books on tape is another option. Although you are not actually reading, you are concentrating and absorbing a wealth of new information. I actually look forward to my commuting time now because I'm always in the middle of a great book on my vehicle's cassette player.

PLAY GAMES AND PUZZLES.

At least one of your weekly brain exercises should involve some form of game or puzzle. Play board or card games that make you think, such as Scrabble, Trivial Pursuit, chess, or bridge. Do crossword puzzles, jigsaw puzzles, word and number games, and brain teasers. There are many books filled with enjoyable, challenging exercises and problems that stimulate your brain. One I particularly recommend is *Brain Builders* by Richard Leviton.

Here are a few examples:

- Count backward from 100 in multiples of four.
- Double a number for as long as you can (2, 4, 8, 16, 32 . . .).
- Choose a special day in your remote past—your sixteenth birthday, for example—and walk yourself through that day, recalling every detail you can: what you were wearing, what you had to eat, and so forth.
- Sketch a picture of an object, but do your drawing upside down.

LEARN A NEW FACT EVERY DAY.
Each new fact you learn will grow new dendrites, so you need to keep feeding your brain new information. Here are some techniques to keep your brain cells on their toes:

- Learn one new vocabulary word each day and then incorporate it into your conversation and writing.
- Memorize a poem, preferably one with several stanzas.
- Pull out an encyclopedia or technical manual and learn how a jet engine works, for example, or how tornadoes are formed.
- Get out an atlas or globe and learn the names of the countries in the world and their capitals.

No matter what kind of new facts you learn, you will be exercising your brain and absorbing new information.

ACQUIRE A NEW SKILL.
Take a class, use a taped instruction series, or get a private tutor. Work on a new language. Learn to play a musical instrument or how to navigate the Internet. Give square dancing a try. (Learning the intricate dance steps is a wonderful way to stimulate new dendrites and improve balance, not to mention that it's good exercise.) Take art lessons. Take up martial arts or yoga. Take a class at a local community college in a subject that has always interested you. A friend of mine, a forty-eight-year-old health food store owner, took a class in automobile maintenance just because she wanted to "understand that hunk of metal" she had been driving for years. Her new knowledge will not only help her maintain her car but will also help her maintain her brain.

BE SOCIAL.
The brain needs stimulation to keep it going, and there is nothing better for the psyche than strong social relationships.

Social interaction is extremely stimulating. Meet new people. Do new things with old friends. Visit museums. Go to movies. Join a book club. Give of yourself. Look into volunteer work at a hospital, preschool, nursing home, church, scout troop, or an organization that interests you. Whatever you do, don't sit around the house, especially if you live alone. Social intercourse is not only a salve for the soul, but it is nourishment for the brain as well.

AGE SAVER:
Exercising Your Body Will Make You Smarter

Did you ever wonder why you feel so recharged after a good workout? Nowhere is the body-mind connection more apparent than when it comes to the effect of exercise on the brain. Exercise increases the amount of oxygen available to the brain by making the heart stronger and able to pump more oxygenated blood. In addition to increasing oxygen stores, exercise creates a natural high. It stimulates the release of endorphins, neurochemicals that actually have an opiatelike effect on the brain. People who exercise think more clearly, feel more alert and energetic, and have a markedly increased sense of well-being.

Researchers at the Veterans' Medical Center in Salt Lake City, Utah, compared the mental function of sedentary older people to those of the same age who were put on an exercise program of fifty minutes of brisk walking three times a week. After four months, participants were tested for reaction time, visual organization, memory, and mental flexibility. Not surprisingly, the exercisers scored higher than the sedentary group in all categories.

The basic exercises outlined above will help boost your brain power for the next ten weeks and if you keep it up, for a lifetime. For those of you who feel that you need that extra edge, however, I recommend some special over-the-counter supplements to boost your brain power. Two are sold over the counter; one supplement, piracetam, is available only by prescription. These should be taken in addition to your Age Loss ODAs.

The supplements that I will now tell you about can be taken individually or together.

Regain Twelve Years of Brain Power with Phosphatidylserine (PS)

As noted earlier, the brain contains a large amount of fatty tissue. One supplement helps replenish a special kind of fat that is important for brain function: phospholipids. Brain cell membranes are made of phospholipids: they not only hold the cell together, but control the entrance and exit of substances to the cells. They are also involved in communication among cells, which is a function of vital importance in the brain.

One of the most plentiful phospholipids in brain tissue is known as "PS," for phosphatidylserine. The role of PS in relaying chemical messages is well established; more than twenty controlled clinical studies have shown its enhancing effects on cell metabolism, neuronal membranes, and neurotransmitters. PS supplements also improve memory. If you are particularly troubled by memory loss, I recommend that you try taking supplemental PS.

One recent study reported in the journal *Neurology*, the bible of brain researchers, involved a group of 149 healthy men and women, from fifty to seventy years of age, who were diagnosed with normal age-associated memory impairment. Participants were given 100 milligrams of PS daily or a placebo for twelve weeks. Those taking the PS noted significant improvements in their ability to recall telephone numbers, names and faces, memorize paragraphs, find misplaced objects, and concentrate while performing tasks. Those who took the placebo showed virtually no change. According to Dr. Thomas H. Crook III, who headed the study, PS supplements brought patients back an average of twelve years in terms of mental function! What this means is that people who took PS performed as well on mental function tests as those twelve years their junior. Perhaps most important, the individuals in the study who had the greatest memory deficits at the start of the study also showed the most significant improvements.

If you feel that you need an extra brain boost, I recommend that you try PS. Begin with 200 to 300 milligrams a day, and then cut down to 100 milligrams daily after eight weeks. PS can be added safely to your supplement plan and taken indefinitely if necessary.

Take the Smart Hormone: Pregnenolone

Hormones are chemicals that exert profound effects on all aspects of human functioning. As we age, the levels of many hormones fall, some of them quite dramatically, and this in turn can affect mental activity. How? The actions of hormones are so widespread and their interactions so vast and complex that they affect every system in the body in some way. They have also been demonstrated to have specific receptor sites and functions within the brain.

Restoring certain hormones to more youthful levels can have a significant impact on brain function. I recommend one hormone in particular: pregnenolone. It has been shown to be the most effective memory-enhancing substance known to date. This hormone, which has only recently been sold over the counter, is produced in the brain and spinal cord, as well as the adrenals. It has a stabilizing effect on memory, mood, and emotion, since it occupies receptors that stimulate the brain as well as others that calm it.

Studies have shown that pregnenolone is an incredibly potent memory enhancer. A study on pregnenolone was conducted fifty years ago with a group of U.S. Army pilots on a flight simulator. Their task was to follow random movements of a model plane using a joystick and rudder pedals for an hour. They were scored on the percentage of time they stayed on target. Obviously, this kind of test requires focused concentration and causes considerable mental fatigue. This was a placebo-controlled study, and the pilots were tested intermittently over two and a half months on three protocols: placebo, 50 milligrams of pregnenolone, and placebo again. During the initial placebo period, scores averaged 25 to 35 percent on target. On pregnenolone, average scores rose from 35 to 50 percent. During the second placebo period, they maintained a higher rate for several days before falling back down to the baseline, indicating that pregnenolone has sustained effects. More recent studies conducted at St. Louis University have also confirmed that pregnenolone can boost memory and concentration in people over fifty.

Pregnenolone does not require a prescription, and there are no known side effects. Take one 50-milligram capsule of pregnenolone daily for ten weeks. If you find that pregnenolone helps you regain your mental edge, you can continue to take it for as long as you need it.

Take the Same "Smart Drug" That I Do: Piracetam

"Smart drugs" are a class of prescription medications designed to boost brain power. One of the most exciting and popular of the new class of "smart" drugs is piracetam. I take it myself, and it is widely used by people who do research on brain function. Piracetam increases the brain's energy reserves, protects it against oxygen starvation, and, as convincingly demonstrated in dozens of studies, improves mental performance.

An early study involved eighteen people, ages fifty or older, with high IQs and "slight but seemingly permanent reduction in their capacity to retain or recall information." These people were completely functional, working in demanding jobs, but they were bothered by the normal age-related mental decline. In this double-blind, placebo-controlled, crossover study, half were given piracetam and half were given a placebo. (Neither the researchers nor the participants knew who was taking the piracetam and who was taking the placebo.) The participants were then given three tests of cognitive function, and the group taking the piracetam scored dramatically higher on all tests. When the placebo group and the piracetam group were "crossed over," or when they switched medications, the group now taking the piracetam had improved scores, while the scores of the group now taking the placebo declined.

I personally have found that piracetam has helped me in two areas: It has increased my powers of concentration and has improved my memory. In particular, I find that I am better able to remember phone numbers, which may not sound like a big deal, but for someone who has to call as many people a day as I do, it can make life a lot easier.

If you are interested in taking piracetam, you will need a prescription from a physician. (For information on where to obtain piracetam, see Resources.)

If you follow my suggestions to boost your brain power, you will feel smarter, sharper, and more alert within ten weeks. If you want to stay that way, I strongly urge you to keep up with your brain exercises. Don't get into a rut: Seek out new mental challenges and keep learning new skills. If you do, you will retain the youthful advantage for your entire life.

Step 6

REVITALIZE YOUR SEX LIFE

Restore your sexual vitality
Enhance your sexual function and performance
Extend your sex life into your 60s, 70s, 80s,
and beyond

RECENTLY, I RECEIVED A tongue-in-cheek note from Shirley, who is the wife of my patient, Bill. Both are in their late 50s. I'd like to share her note with you.

> Dear Dr. Whitaker:
>
> I certainly do appreciate and enjoy what you have done for my husband, Bill. I don't want to complain, but we have had sex 18 times in the last 17 days, and I am exhausted. Can you please cut back on my husband's medication?
>
> Yours truly,
> Shirley J.

I love to receive letters like Shirley's because they confirm my belief that an active and enjoyable sex life is possible at any age. When Shirley and Bill first came to see me last year, they had a hard time believing my first rule of the Age Loss Program: It's never too late to benefit from the Whitaker Age

Loss Program. They, like so many couples who are middle-aged and older, believed that their sex life was over. They did not even consider the possibility that it could be revived. So hopeless did they consider the situation that Bill did not even bother to tell me about it . . . until I asked.

Bill had come to the Whitaker Wellness Institute for treatment of high cholesterol. In the course of his physical exam I asked him about sex. "Nonexistent" was his curt reply. When I pressed the subject, Bill reluctantly told me that he and Shirley used to enjoy great sex, but because of his inability to perform, they had not had sex for over a year. As a result, Shirley felt rejected, and their marriage started feeling the stress. I prescribed a regimen of supplements, foods, and exercise that enabled Bill to regain his ability to have and enjoy sex. Judging from Shirley's letter, my program worked even better than we had hoped!

Shirley and Bill are not atypical. The most common but least talked about problems of midlife are those related to sexual function and enjoyment. Although sex is discussed with great frankness in our society, sexual problems are not. Ironically, I think that all this so-called openness about sex actually prevents people from bringing their problems to the attention of their doctors. Sex is presented so explicitly in the media that we all tend to think that everyone around us is having great sex and that if we are not, we must be inadequate. The result is that people suffer in silence and isolation, and what's worse, they suffer needlessly.

This is why I don't wait for my patients to tell me about their sex problems. I ask them directly.

My patients tend to be very relieved to hear that they are not alone and that many people after age forty do experience at least some problems related to sexual performance and function. They are even more relieved to find out that nearly all their problems can be solved. In fact, the best news is that most problems related to sex can be prevented in the first place. By following my ten-week program you will be on your way toward revitalizing your sex life. Each step of my Age Loss Program—from the use of supplements to the food plan to the workout routines—will help prevent and correct the common problems that can interfere with sexual enjoyment. Step 6 includes some additional ways to maintain and enhance your sex life.

Neither gender, by the way, has a monopoly on sexual problems. As you might expect, however, men and women experience them very differently, and therefore my approach varies accordingly. I have broken this approach into two parts, one for men and one for women.

ALL ABOUT MEN

Until recently, doctors tended to recommend psychological counseling when men over forty complained of sexual problems. Although the advice was well intended, the therapy was not very effective in many cases. Today we know that most of the performance problems experienced by men originate not in the head but in other parts of the body.

I do not want to suggest that male sexual problems do not exact an emotional toll. They most certainly do. Indeed, I have found that when men lose confidence in their ability to perform sexually, they lose confidence in their ability to do many other things. This can be a blow to their egos and to their sense of independence. Sexual prowess is linked to youth, strength, and continuity. When we lose it, we feel we are no longer "in the game" and may even feel useless and expendable. Counseling may help us cope with those feelings, and that is fine—but it is not enough. We also need to treat the underlying causes of sexual problems. Let me assure you, most are eminently treatable, but it is important to understand what happens to men as they age and how it affects male sexual function.

The problem is partly hormonal. We all know that at midlife, women experience a decline in their levels of certain sex hormones and that this decline leads to menopause. What most people don't realize is that men also experience midlife changes in hormone production. Although these changes are not as sudden or as dramatic as those experienced by women, at about age forty most men notice that their bodies are beginning to behave differently. This is largely due to a decline in the production of testosterone, the "male" hormone that is responsible for sex drive and that plays an important role in sexual function. About 30 percent of all men end up with abnormally low levels of testosterone and experience depression, lethargy, loss of muscle mass, and loss of libido.

Even men who don't fall into this 30 percent category will notice subtle changes. The most evident is that they don't get erections as often, as easily, or as rigidly as they did when younger. Although men over forty may experience an occasional "off day," this does not mean they are impotent or that their sex lives are finished. Nothing could be further from the truth.

Only a small number of men actually suffer from complete impotence—that is, they are unable to have satisfying sexual activity because of *chronic* erection problems. At age forty, 5 percent of men are completely impotent, but by age seventy, that number climbs to 15 percent. I'm not telling you this to frighten you but to assure you that sexual impotence can be prevented. In reality, most of the serious problems that hamper sexual activity have little to do with normal aging, and everything to do with years of neglect of your body and health. As I will explain, simple changes in lifestyle can have an enormously positive effect on a man's sex life and can even reverse many problems that were once considered intractable.

Indeed, for men who already have problems, I have even better news: Some new high-tech solutions can work absolute miracles.

The Age Loss Program Will Help You Maintain Your Sexual Vigor

If you follow my Age Loss Program, you should be able to maintain your sexual vigor and vitality well into the last decades of life. I feel comfortable in making this assertion because I know that most cases of impotence are caused not by organic problems but by unhealthy eating, drinking, and smoking habits. You already know that these "age accelerators," which are responsible for hardening of the arteries, high blood pressure, and diabetes, will kill you. But did you know that long before they kill you they will kill your sex life? Consider the following:

- In order to maintain an erection, blood must flow freely to the penis through the penile artery. If the penile artery becomes clogged, getting and maintaining an erection becomes difficult or impossible. About half of all cases of impotence are due to atherosclerosis of the penile artery!
- High blood pressure can cause damage to arteries, including the penile artery.
- Ninety percent of all heavy smokers will suffer damage to the penile artery. (I have often wondered what would happen if those cigarette warning labels read: "Cigarettes can make you impotent." I wonder how many men would continue to smoke! I wonder how many teenagers would start!)
- Ironically, drug therapies for atherosclerosis and high blood pressure do not solve the problem of sexual dysfunction but, rather, tend to compound it, because one of their most common (and commonly complained of) side effects is impotence.

My Age Loss Program, especially my Age Loss ODAs and food plan, will help *prevent* and even reverse the underlying conditions that give rise to impotence. The program's heart-friendly lifestyle will keep your arteries young and your blood flowing freely, and will prevent or control conditions such as diabetes that can destroy sexual desire and function.

Stress and Sex

In addition to keeping your body in condition for good sex, the Age Loss Program will also help keep you in the right frame of mind. Although most problems related to sexual function have a physical component, in many cases stress is a contributing factor. In Step 8 I describe in detail how the stress response adversely affects every cell of our physical being. In fact, stress hormones can inflict significant damage on body tissues, causing the very conditions that can lead to sexual dysfunction. Stress hormones also profoundly affect the brain and can "shut down" production of sex hormones, which are essential for libido.

Unfortunately, many of us who feel stressed seek comfort through unhealthy outlets such as excessive alcohol con-sumption—which, contrary to popular myth, is actually a sexual downer. Although a small amount of alcohol may ap-pear to stimulate sex drive by reducing inhibitions, in reality alcohol is very *unsexy*. More than two alcoholic drinks daily can decrease testosterone production and interfere with sex drive and the ability to have an erection. Many men have found that by simply cutting back on alcohol consumption, they can reinvigorate their sex lives.

It goes without saying that when you are faced with chronic and relentless stress, romance is the last thing on your mind. (For more information on how to control stress before it controls you, see page 216.)

And finally, as I tell my patients, the greatest aphrodisiac of all is good physical and mental health. When you feel and look better, you also feel sexier. And the Age Loss Program will help you do both.

AGE SAVER: In the Morning It Is up and at 'Em

Many men may awaken with an erection even if they have difficulty getting one at night. If you feel amorous in the morning, take advantage of the situation. Many couples find that sex is better when they are feeling morning fresh and ready to greet the day.

Sex and the Prostate

One of the major concerns of men over forty is the health of their prostate gland. Benign prostate hypertrophy, or BPH, is very common among middle-aged men. It is not cancer nor is it serious, but it can be uncomfortable and can make sex uncomfortable. There are many things you can do to prevent or postpone the onset of BPH. To understand the cure, let's examine the underlying cause.

The prostate is a small, walnut-shaped gland that surrounds the part of the urethra that is located under the bladder. Urine passes via the urethra from the bladder through the prostate and out the penis. Just below the prostate and surrounding the urethra is the urethral sphincter, which is contracted to stop urine flow.

At around age forty, the prostate gland undergoes a growth spurt that is the result of a hormonal chain reaction: Levels of the hormone prolactin rise, stimulating the activity of an enzyme called 5-alpha-reductase, which in turn converts testosterone into a more potent and problematic form: dihydrotestosterone.

Dihydrotestosterone is an androgen, which means that it produces male characteristics and is essential for the development of the male fetus. When it kicks in again in middle age, however, it can stimulate the growth of the prostate. When the prostate grows, it chokes off the urethra, interfering with urine flow and forcing the bladder to work harder to expel urine. This causes the muscles of the bladder to strengthen and become so sensitive that even small amounts of urine in the bladder cause the feeling of an urgent need to urinate. The problem is particularly acute at night when there are fewer distractions to interfere with the bladder's signals to the brain.

As BPH progresses, it can cause the problems known as "hesitancy" (the condition that leaves you standing there waiting . . . and waiting . . . for seconds or even minutes until urine starts to flow); "intermittency" (the annoying series of contractions that start and stop flow but never fully empty the bladder); and complete obstruction of flow (which can lead to an infection that is not only painful and annoying but life threatening).

Another related condition is prostatitis or inflammation of the prostate, which can put a damper on your sex life. Robert W. is a case in point. A fifty-five-year-old construction supervisor with a dislike for doctors, he consulted me only because his wife talked him into it. He complained that he had to get up several times a night to go to the bathroom, slept fitfully, and sometimes couldn't get back to sleep at all. Urinating was painful to him, as was intercourse. Robert's biggest fear was that he would have to put up with this problem for the rest of his life.

Fortunately, he didn't have to. At the Whitaker Wellness Institute we have had terrific results treating and preventing prostate disorders through diet and inexpensive, readily available supplements that are sold over the counter and are free of side effects. I believe that every man over forty should use these supplements to guard against prostate problems. If you are already being treated for a prostate problem, I recommend that you find a physician who will work with you to incorporate these natural therapies into your treatment. The esteemed *Journal of Urology* recently reported that more and more "traditional" urologists are turning to natural remedies because they believe they work as well as, if not better than, some of the standard therapies.

And if you are experiencing symptoms such as frequent urination, especially at night, burning during urination, an inability to urinate, or stopping and starting during urination, you should see your doctor. You need to rule out other problems before you begin your treatment.

Supplements and Foods to Protect You

Many of the supplements already included in the Age Loss ODAs will help prevent prostate problems and maintain sexual vitality. For example, zinc (which should be included in your high-potency multivitamin) is absolutely essential for male sexual health. Make sure you are taking 30 milligrams of zinc daily. If 30 milligrams are not included in your multivitamin, you need to take an additional zinc supplement.

Marginal zinc deficiency is widespread in the United States, especially among middle-aged and older men. There is a higher concentration of zinc in the prostate than anywhere else in the body and many researchers suspect that a lack of zinc contributes to BPH and other problems related to the male reproductive system, such as low sperm count.

To prevent these problems I also recommend that men eat a diet rich in zinc, foods that include oysters (cooked, never raw!), wheat germ, wheat bran, legumes, and raw pumpkin seeds, which are an old folk remedy for BPH. I have seen men make great improvement simply by eating one-fourth to one-half cup of them daily. Oysters have been touted as a natural aphrodisiac for centuries, and I believe their reputation derives from their zinc content and their effect on prostate health.

Soy foods (such as tofu and soy-based veggie burgers) are rich in zinc and are also a veritable pharmacy of phytochemicals which can deactivate the process that causes the prostate to grow. There is also good evidence that these same phytochemicals can prevent the spread of prostate cancer. Here's a riddle with an important lesson: The incidence of prostate cancer is the same for men in the United States and Japan, yet American men are five times more likely to die of prostate cancer than are Japanese men. The reason appears to be related to the soy-rich diet of Japanese men, who eat ten times more soy food than American men.

Hundreds of studies have documented that several of the phytochemicals found in soy foods, including genistein and daidzein, can stop the growth of prostate cancer cells. The great danger of prostate cancer is that it will spread to other organ systems. If the cancer remains confined to the prostate, it will not interfere with a man's normal life span. The same hormones that trigger BPH can also stimulate the growth of hormone-dependent tumors in the prostate. Dampening the destructive effect of these hormones will therefore not only help prevent BPH but will also prevent the spread of prostate cancer. So I urge you to add soy foods to your diet, as recommended in Step 2.

Another supplement that you are already taking if you are following the Age Loss ODAs is ginkgo biloba, an herbal antioxidant that can boost sexual function in men whose erection problems are due to impairment of blood flow. In one study, fifty impotent men were given 240 milligrams of ginkgo biloba extract daily for nine months. Some of the men were also given injections of the drug papaverine, a muscle stimulant that can boost erections. The results? The ginkgo biloba supplements greatly improved erections in both groups of men, *whether or not they had received the additional injections of papaverine.* In an earlier study, ginkgo biloba had been shown to be effective in restoring erections in men who did not respond to papaverine. Ginkgo biloba is hardly a new or untested treatment. It has been used for thousands of years by Asian healers and is safe, nontoxic, and inexpensive. This is one herb that everyone should take! (The Age Loss ODA for ginkgo biloba is 120 milligrams daily.)

There are a few supplements not included in the Age Loss ODAs that I highly recommend you take to revitalize your sex life.

RX FOR MEN: ADD THESE SEXUALLY REVITALIZING SUPPLEMENTS TO YOUR SUPPLEMENT PLAN

Saw Palmetto Berry Extract

Long touted as an aphrodisiac and used by Native Americans, the saw palmetto herb is a safe, nontoxic, and effective way to prevent and treat BPH. Saw palmetto berry extract gets to the root of BPH by inhibiting the activity of the enzyme that converts good testosterone into dihydrotestosterone.

Saw palmetto is widely used throughout Europe to treat prostate problems and is the treatment of choice in Germany and France. Saw palmetto has been carefully studied in laboratories and hospitals around the world, and more than a dozen clinical studies have been done on its effectiveness.

At the Whitaker Wellness Institute we regularly prescribe saw palmetto to any man over forty, and to patients who have

BPH. We typically see marked improvement within four to six weeks. Therefore, if you are over forty or are suffering from BPH, I recommend that you take 160 milligrams daily of saw palmetto extract. (Saw palmetto is also sold under the botanical name of *serenoa repens.*)

L-Arginine for Better Erections

If you are having difficulty maintaining an erection long enough to have satisfactory sex, I suggest that you try the amino acid L-arginine, which is sold at health food stores and pharmacies. L-arginine increases blood flow to the penis, which can result in harder erections with more staying power and frequency. L-arginine is a powder that can be mixed in water or juice. As a sexual aid, take 3 to 6 grams of L-arginine forty-five minutes before sex. (Start out with 3 grams, and if that doesn't work, increase your dose the next time you try it by 1 gram until you reach the full 6 grams.) L-arginine doesn't work for everybody, but many men have told me that it has made a real difference in their ability to enjoy sex.

AGE SAVER: Pump those muscles!

People who exercise have more sex, much more sex, than people who don't. In a study of 160 master swimmers between the ages of forty and eighty, researchers found that those who exercised the most had sex lives that were typical of people twenty to forty years their junior!

For most men these supplements and simple remedies will enhance sexual function and prevent the kinds of problems that interfere with sexual enjoyment. If these over-the-counter treatments don't work for you, however, other treatments are available by prescription—namely, testosterone, which many experts predict will become as commonplace for men as estrogen replacement therapy is for women, and yohimbine, the only prescriptive drug recognized as a treatment for impotence. The descriptions below will familiarize you with these treatments so you can consult with your doctor.

By Rx Only:
Testosterone Replacement Therapy for Men

As noted earlier, about one-third of all men over forty may have low testosterone levels. When a male patient complains of either low sex drive, fatigue, weakness, or difficulty getting or maintaining an erection, one of the first things I check is his blood level of the male hormone testosterone. If his testosterone level is low, I prescribe supplemental testosterone.

Testosterone is produced by the adrenal glands (located on top of the kidneys) and the testes, and is the primary regulator of the male reproductive system. In boys, testosterone controls the growth of the reproductive organs and the development of secondary male characteristics, such as deepening of the voice and the growth of body hair. In men (and in women, as I will explain later), testosterone is the hormone that controls sex drive.

Although testosterone is the hormone that turns on the libido, its effect on a man's ability to perform sexually is somewhat less defined. Clearly, testosterone is involved in sexual response and function—it is instrumental in the production of sperm and the ability to maintain an erection—but it cannot do the job alone. In fact, when synthetic testosterone first became available, it was routinely used as a treatment for erection problems, and often with disappointing results.

We now know that testosterone replacement will not cure all erectile problems, especially if these problems are caused by other health problems such as atherosclerosis. But I have found that in many cases, testosterone replacement is nothing short of miraculous. If there are no other underlying health problems hampering a man's ability to have an erection, testosterone therapy may be all that is needed to restore normal sexual function.

Testosterone is essential for male health and well-being. It is an anabolic hormone, which means that it is critical for tissue building and heavily involved in the making of muscle. Testosterone is also a psychic energizer and a natural mood elevator that infuses men with an enthusiasm for life.

Low levels of testosterone will result in a loss of sex drive, muscle strength, lack of energy, and mild depression. The problem is that too many people dismiss these symptoms as part of the normal aging process. That is simply not the case. There is nothing normal about not feeling healthy, alive, and vital at any age. If you have these symptoms, I recommend that you find a doctor who will take your symptoms seriously and test your testosterone levels.

From age twenty on, blood levels of testosterone begin to decline in men, and by forty or fifty some men may have levels that are well below normal. Testosterone levels vary widely from man to man, and can be as low as 300 ng./dl or as high as 1,200 ng./dl. Ideally, testosterone levels should be between 900 and 1,200 ng./dl. If a patient's total blood levels of testosterone are below this ideal, I usually recommend supplementation. Testosterone is available in many different forms, including gels, creams, pellets that are surgically inserted under the skin, and a transdermal patch that is worn on the skin, but I find that weekly injections of testosterone ciprionate (100 milligrams weekly) to be the most effective. For convenience' sake I teach my patients (or their spouses) to administer the injections in their own homes.

I recommend that any man over forty who is suffering from low sex drive, fatigue, and difficulty getting or maintaining an erection should make an appointment with his doctor to check his testosterone level. You may simply need to supplement testosterone to regain your sex drive and eliminate—or prevent—other problems.

Men who are taking testosterone also need to be monitored by their physicians for potential side effects. Although testosterone does not cause prostate cancer, it could promote the growth of an existing tumor, so men with prostate cancer or a history of prostate cancer treatment should not take it.

Yohimbine: An FDA-Approved Aphrodisiac

For centuries, natural healers have used the bark of the African yohimbe tree as an aphrodisiac. A drug derived from yohimbe, yohimbine hydrochloride, is the only drug approved by the FDA for enhancing sexual desire. Yohimbine not only revs up libido but increases the blood flow to the penis, making it easier to get and maintain erections. In a recent Canadian study, forty-eight men who had erection problems were given either yohimbine or a placebo over a ten-week period. Positive results were reported by 46 percent of the men taking yohimbine; the men taking the placebo reported scant improvement.

Yohimbine is not for everyone, however, and should be taken under a doctor's supervision. Yohimbine can cause fluctuations in blood pressure, dizziness, and even anxiety attacks in some people, and can also interact with commonly used medications such as antidepressants. People with heart disease or kidney problems should definitely not take it, so make sure that your doctor knows your medical history.

A weaker version of yohimbine, yohimbe, is sold over the counter in health food stores, but I would not advise you to take it unless you first consult your doctor. The product I recommend is Male Fuel manufactured by Twin Labs; it contains 800 milligrams of yohimbe bark extract as well as other ingredients, including zinc, ginkgo biloba, and L-arginine. Patients with libido or mild erectile problems have reported some terrific results after taking Male Fuel, and for some it seems to be pure magic. Even in its weakened form, however, yohimbe has the potential to cause side effects similar to yohimbine, so please talk to your doctor to make sure that you do not have any medical conditions that can be aggravated by this herb.

Numerous other treatments for sexual dysfunction in men are available by prescription, such as penile injections, which is a simple way to remedy erection problems. The penile injection delivers a chemical relaxant directly into the side of the penis via a very thin needle; despite the sensitivity of the area, it causes minimal discomfort. I have prescribed this method to hundreds of patients, with good results. The point is that if you have a problem that cannot be remedied by simple measures, I urge you to talk to your physician.

FOR WOMEN ONLY

I'm having the best sex I've had in my entire life.

SELMA M., 73

Although the midlife hormonal changes that women experience are far more sudden and dramatic than the hormonal changes experienced by men, women have a decided advantage over men: They have fewer sexual problems, and the problems they have tend to be easy to remedy. Based on the experience of my patients, many women in their middle years

188

and older can have thoroughly fulfilling sex lives. Women in their 50s, 60s, and 70s tell me that they regard these years as the best of their lives and that they feel as if they are in their sexual prime. Most are liberated from their child-rearing responsibilities, some are relieved from job and career burdens, and their life experience has given them a new sense of confidence. I truly believe that if a woman takes care of her health and vitality, there is no reason that she cannot look forward to an active and enjoyable sex life indefinitely.

When women do encounter sexual obstacles, it is usually due to midlife changes associated with menopause. At around age fifty, women become menopausal or experience their last menstrual cycle. As most readers know, menopause is caused by a decline in two key hormones: estrogen and progesterone. These are produced in women by the ovaries and the adrenal glands. After age thirty the production of these hormones begins slowly to decline; the decline is fast and furious in their late 40s and early 50s. As the ovaries cease functioning, they no longer produce estrogen, and the level of estrogen drops precipitously. Progesterone production virtually shuts down.

The loss of these key female hormones can produce a variety of symptoms, affecting some women more acutely than others. Some women will feel no change and will go on without missing a beat. Others will experience unpleasant symptoms, including hot flashes, headaches, fatigue, insomnia, depression, and, not surprisingly given these other symptoms, loss of libido. The decline in estrogen and progesterone can also leave women vulnerable to heart disease, osteoporosis, memory loss, and other health problems. At one time doctors considered these symptoms normal, but today no physician worth his or her salt will allow a patient to suffer from menopausal discomfort. Several simple remedies can help normalize hormone levels, reverse the unpleasant symptoms, and restore libido.

Although women never lose their ability to engage in

sexual activity, the decline in key sex hormones that they experience may make sex uncomfortable. For example, low estrogen levels may cause vaginal dryness and thinning of the vaginal walls. Rest assured, none of these minor problems caused by menopause should interfere with a woman's ability or desire to have sex. They can all be solved quickly, simply, and safely.

AGE SAVER: The Joy of Soy

If menopausal symptoms are interfering with sexual enjoyment, I urge you to eat more soy foods, because they are loaded with natural plant estrogens. Eating three to four ounces of tofu or drinking a cup of soy milk daily can give you an estrogen boost that will significantly reduce vaginal dryness and make sex more pleasurable.

Estrogen Replacement Therapy: By Prescription Only

If a woman is having severe menopausal symptoms, I prescribe estrogen replacement therapy, which will relieve these symptoms within a matter of weeks. When I utter the words "estrogen replacement therapy," however, some of my patients react with alarm. They typically express concern that estrogen may increase their risk of developing breast and other cancers. This is not so. But there is a great deal of misunderstanding about estrogen, so let me take this opportunity to set the record straight.

First and foremost: Estrogen does *not* cause cancer. Estrogen can stimulate the growth of an existing tumor, however, especially those in the breast that are hormone dependent. Numerous studies have examined the link between estrogen and breast cancer, and the results are far from conclusive. On the other hand, hundreds of studies have documented that estrogen users enjoy a decided advantage over nonusers in many ways. We know, for example, that estrogen users are less likely to get Alzheimer's disease, osteoporosis, and heart disease.

Second: Not all estrogen is the same. The type of estrogen that I prescribe to my patients is not only safe but actually protects against breast cancer. Three different types of estrogen are produced by the female body: estrone, estradiol, and estriol. Estrone is the strongest, estradiol is somewhat weaker, and estriol is the weakest. Stronger estrogens are believed to be more apt to stimulate tumor growth, and therefore I steer away from them.

No doubt you have heard the pros and cons of using estrogen. The debate over its use has been fueled by the fact that the estrogen most commonly used in hormone replacement therapy is not the same in chemical structure as the estrogen produced by women. Rather, it is a blend of ten different types of estrogen found in the urine of pregnant mares (hence the name "Premarin") and is stronger than the estrogen produced naturally in a woman's body. I do not prescribe Premarin for my patients. Instead, I prescribe a mix of two natural estrogens that are identical in chemical structure to the estrogen produced by women.

The estrogen I use in my practice is called Bi-Estrogen; as its name suggests, it is a combination of two estrogens. Bi-Estrogen is 80 percent estriol (the weakest estrogen produced by women) and 20 percent estradiol. Because Bi-estrogen contains higher levels of estriol than any other estrogen, I believe that this formula is the best. Studies have shown that estriol has a protective effect against breast cancer, and in contrast to stronger estrogens, it appears to inhibit tumor growth. In addition, studies have also shown that women with breast cancer have lower than normal levels of estriol and that the converse is also true. Asian women and vegetarians, who have a much lower than normal risk of breast cancer, have higher levels of estriol.

The reason that natural estrogen is not more frequently prescribed is again because it cannot be patented and there is no pharmaceutical company championing its cause or willing to shell out hundreds of millions of dollars to obtain FDA approval. Drug salesmen don't push it, so many doctors don't even know about it. In the Resource section of this book I suggest how you can identify a doctor who will prescribe natural estrogen and a compounding pharmacist who will prepare it. For those of you who are already on estrogen replacement therapy, you may want to talk to your doctor about switching to natural estrogen.

Progesterone

Any woman who takes estrogen must also take progesterone to protect against uterine cancer; at exception are women who have had hysterectomies (the removal of the uterus). Estrogen can stimulate the growth of the uterine lining, which can increase the risk of uterine cancer. If your doctor puts you on estrogen replacement therapy, he most likely will put you on progesterone, too. I prescribe topical progesterone creams for my patients who are taking natural estrogen, which is described below.

And even if you do not take estrogen, most menopausal women will benefit from taking natural progesterone, a mood enhancer that can restore a sluggish libido.

Natural Progesterone: An Over-the-Counter Solution to Rev Up Your Sex Drive

Recently I treated a fifty-year-old woman, Karen, who had just become menopausal. When I asked her how she was feeling, she replied that it wasn't what she was feeling that worried her, it was what she wasn't feeling. What she wasn't feeling was sexy. She said that she was no longer able to summon up the energy or the desire to have sex.

Based on Karen's symptoms, I recommended natural progesterone cream, a safe over-the-counter remedy derived from yams and soybeans that is sold by health food stores and pharmacies. If a woman is suffering from low sex drive, I generally recommend progesterone supplementation as a first step.

I call progesterone the "feel good" hormone for women because it is most plentiful at the times in a woman's life when she is either at her happiest or most interested in sex. Progesterone is produced in high amounts during pregnancy, when women typically report feelings of euphoria or enhanced feelings of well-being. Progesterone levels also rise in a woman's body during the week following ovulation, the point in the monthly cycle when women are most fertile and when many women experience a surge in sexual interest. Since menopausal women produce virtually no progesterone, it stands to reason that replenishing progesterone would have a beneficial effect on a woman's sense of well-being and sex drive.

Within a month after starting on progesterone, Karen not only reported an increase in libido but also said that she generally felt healthier and more energetic. The phrase that she used is one that so many women use to describe the effect of natural progesterone: "I feel more like myself." Helping a woman feel more like herself is precisely the goal of the treatment and the goal of the Age Loss Program.

Progesterone cream is very easy to use. Postmenopausal women should apply one-fourth to one-half teaspoon of cream twice daily. It is applied to the soft skin of the abdomen, inner thighs, inner arms, or face. I recommend switching areas of application for more effective absorption. (In other words, do the arms and thighs in the morning, and the face and abdomen at night.)

There are several good natural progesterone creams, which are sold at most pharmacies. You can also obtain high-quality progesterone cream from a compounding pharmacist.

If you do not want to use cream, natural progesterone is available in capsules. I typically recommend between 100 and 200 milligrams daily of oral progesterone if you are not using the cream. The form of oral progesterone that I use in my practice is called micronized progesterone. "Micronized" means that it is broken up into tiny particles that are easily absorbed.

Do not confuse *natural progesterone* with *synthetic progestins*, the form of progesterone widely prescribed by physicians as part of hormone replacement therapy for menopause. Many women find that progestins cause unpleasant side effects, including mood swings, loss of libido, headache, and bloating, the very symptoms that women are trying to cure! The progesterone creams and supplements that I recommend should not have any unpleasant side effects.

By Prescription Only: Testosterone for Women

Although progesterone replacement will work beautifully for most women, some need an extra push to restore sex drive and desire. In these cases I may prescribe testosterone, a hormone that can be a real boon to women although it is more widely known for its effect on men. You may be surprised to learn that testosterone is the hormone that controls the sex drive in women as well as in men and is produced in the bodies of both women and men. A woman who is low on testosterone will feel tired, depressed, and have a marked disinterest in sex.

Testosterone is not only important for a woman's emotional well-being but it is vital for normal physical development. Testosterone is produced in both the ovaries and the adrenal glands of women, although in much smaller amounts than it is produced in men. Women's blood levels of testosterone range between 15 and 100 ng./dl; for men the range is 300 ng./dl to 1,200 ng./dl.

Although most people think of estrogen as the hormone that controls sexual reproduction in women, in reality, puberty and the onset of menstruation are triggered by a sharp increase in testosterone and another hormone called DHEA. This is known as the adrenarch. In women, testosterone levels fluctuate throughout the menstrual cycle and rise prior to ovulation. By age forty women produce far less testosterone than they did at age twenty, and by menopause they may produce none. As in men, the drop in testosterone varies from woman to woman, and some may feel it more acutely than others.

Until recently we really did not know much about the important role that testosterone plays in maintaining a woman's interest in sex. Much of what we know today is due to the work of Dr. Barbara Sherwin, a psychologist at McGill University in Montreal, who more than a decade ago began research on women and testosterone. As part of her research, Dr. Sherwin tested the effect of using either estrogen alone or a combination of estrogen and testosterone on young women who had undergone premature menopause due to hysterectomy. Since testosterone is primarily made in the ovaries, these women experienced a decline in testosterone not dissimilar to women who undergo menopause naturally. Dr. Sherwin's studies revealed that women who took both the estrogen and the testosterone were more interested in sex, enjoyed sex more and even had more orgasms than those who took estrogen alone.

That is why when a postmenopausal woman complains of a loss of libido, I consider testosterone replacement therapy. In fact, in my practice I have prescribed testosterone to both husbands and wives. The women receive a much smaller dose of testosterone (2.5 milligrams three times a week) in the form of a lozenge that can be dissolved under the tongue. Most women say they feel the effects of this treatment within five days, and the results have been excellent.

Many women express concern that testosterone will produce masculine side effects, such as excess hair growth or a deepening of their voice. Let me assure you that the appropriately small amount of testosterone prescribed for a woman should not produce any untoward side effects. That said, one caveat is in order: Some studies have shown that testosterone replacement therapy can lower HDL, or good cholesterol, in women. Low HDL is a risk factor for heart disease. If a woman has a history of heart disease or low HDL, she should not take testosterone. And every woman who is taking testosterone should have her cholesterol tested each year to make sure she is not losing too much of the good HDL.

Women can also take testosterone via injection or, in some cases, by slow-release subcutaneous skin pellets implanted under the skin. Testosterone creams and gels are also available from compounding pharmacists and may be included in preparations containing estrogen and progesterone.

Although it is becoming more common, testosterone replacement therapy for women is still a fairly recent development, and some doctors may be unfamiliar with the protocol. The Resource section gives information on how to find a doctor who is knowledgeable in the use of testosterone for women.

Good health is the ultimate aphrodisiac for both men and women. The best way to revitalize your sex life is to take the necessary steps to reclaim and safeguard your health. Sex is a life-affirming and life-enhancing activity for all people regardless of age. We should not forgo the best part of life simply because we are getting older. Maintaining good and close relationships is what sustains us through life and makes life worth living. It is what the Age Loss Program is all about.

Step 7

REJUVENATE WHILE YOU SLEEP

Restore youthful sleep patterns
Wake up feeling refreshed and renewed
Enjoy the extraordinary benefits of a good night's sleep

THROUGHOUT THIS BOOK I have recommended several state-of-the art techniques to shed those extra years. Now I am going to discuss one of the most basic and effective ways to turn back the clock. In a word: *sleep.*

Improving the quality of your sleep is a critical part of the Age Loss Program. For obvious reasons a well-rested mind and body can greet the challenges of life more effectively. But there's more to sleep than most people realize.

For the next ten weeks I want you to think of a good night's sleep as a mini vacation. Sleep provides you with an opportunity to recharge and reinvigorate every system in the body; it gives you the ability to cope with stress and ward off infection. Sleep gives your body and mind time to regroup, rejuvenate, and basically rediscover the resilience that can help keep you feeling and looking young. You cannot achieve the goal of shedding ten years in ten weeks unless you learn how to tap the amazing power of sleep.

ARE YOU GETTING ENOUGH SLEEP?

Before I discuss how to improve the *quality* of your sleep, we need to address an important issue: Are you getting enough sleep? Most people don't know how to answer this question. Frankly, the answer should vary from person to person. Perhaps the best way to find the answer is to ask yourself another question: Do you feel alert and reinvigorated in the morning? If not, you are probably not getting enough sleep.

Lack of sleep is a major problem for many people. Americans spend 20 percent less time sleeping than we did a hundred years ago. This is not surprising, considering the fact that we live in a world that never sleeps. At the turn of the century, people slept from dusk until dawn, averaging about nine and a half hours a night. Today most people sleep on average seven and a half hours a night, and for many people that's not enough. Unlike our great-grandparents who had few distractions after dark, when the sun goes down our world lights up. Late-night television, twenty-four-hour supermarkets, and computers that never rest are robbing us of precious hours we should be sleeping.

Stress is another reason that so many of us have difficulty sleeping. As modern life becomes more complicated, more and more people suffer from conditions such as depression and anxiety that can keep them up tossing and turning at night. And it should not surprise you to know that age affects our sleep patterns. From age forty on, physiological changes make people especially vulnerable to disruptive sleep patterns. This is both frustrating and hard on your body.

The net result is that many of us are walking around tired, irritable, and frustrated. In other words, we feel "out of whack." More troubling still, this lack of sleep increases our susceptibility to infections and stress-related illnesses, and it vastly accelerates the aging process.

The good news is that *we don't have to take it anymore.* In Step 8 I will teach you how you can use sleep as a tool of rejuvenation. I will show you how simple it is to consistently get a great night's sleep and how you can wake up every morning feeling refreshed and renewed.

First, let's take a look at what a good night's sleep actually is and why it is so important to the Age Loss Program.

Sleep: A Time of Renewal

A restful night is one in which we continuously cycle in and out of the various stages of sleep with few or no interruptions. How long we sleep or the amount of time we spend in each stage is simply not as important as the peacefulness of our slumber.

There are two kinds of sleep: REM (rapid eye movement) sleep and non-REM. Each night we have four to six sleep cycles, each consisting of REM and non-REM sleep. During REM sleep we dream; during non-REM sleep we don't. Non-REM sleep comes in two forms. The most frequent form is called Stage 2, and the much deeper version is called Delta sleep or Stages 3 and 4.

Delta sleep is the phase that allows the body to recover and a time when body systems can relax. At the onset of Delta sleep the largest spurt of growth hormone is released in the entire twenty-four-hour cycle. As we age, we produce less growth hormone, and as a result our muscles weaken and we lose bone. If we do not get enough Delta sleep, we disrupt our production of growth hormone and deny ourselves a powerful tool for rejuvenation.

REM sleep, on the other hand, seems to be more involved

with mood and mental function. If you don't have sufficient REM sleep at night, it's difficult to focus or think clearly in the morning. Researchers have found that people deprived of REM sleep become agitated, confused, and forgetful, sometimes bordering on hallucinating. A chronic lack of REM sleep is also associated with a higher risk of psychological problems.

A good night's sleep allows our body and mind to rest and refuel. Our body systems wind down while we are sleeping. Our heart and respiratory rates markedly decrease, and blood pressure begins to drop. Our metabolism, the process by which our body uses energy, switches into low gear, and our body temperature drops. During sleep we are far less demanding on our organ systems than when we are awake; it is the time when our body's cells can concentrate on repairing themselves and create new healthy cells.

A restless night's sleep means that your body doesn't have the chance to rest and sufficiently rejuvenate.

WHY CAN'T YOU SLEEP?

To find the cure, you must pinpoint the problem. At least half of all sleep problems are caused by common psychological factors, including anxiety, depression, marital difficulties, grief, or job concerns. These problems are not always easy to self-diagnose, but it stands to reason that if you're under a great deal of stress during the day, it can spill over into the night.

Yet too many of us push our worries aside rather than confront them. If you are having difficulty sleeping, falling asleep, or sleeping through the night and can't pinpoint the cause, do some soul searching. Have you recently been rejected in an important personal relationship? Are you worried about someone's health or even your own? Do you have financial problems? Remember, even *good* changes in your life can be stressful. Have you recently switched jobs? Are you in the middle of a move? Are you embarking on a new relationship?

Don't get me wrong. I don't want to call attention to your problems, I simply want to make you aware of what is causing your stress so that you can learn to put it out of your mind, at least at night.

Over the next ten weeks, I would like you to try to keep your evenings as *worry free* as possible. Once you realize that what is on your mind is disrupting your sleep, I want you to try the following exercises.

Take a Worry Break

Find thirty minutes during the late afternoon to take a "worry break." Sit down quietly. Worry. Do it intensely. Think about what is bothering you and how you can make the situation better. Some people find that actually writing down the problem and listing possible solutions can be beneficial. If there is something you can do to resolve a problem, do it or at least formulate a plan of action. Then put worrying aside until the next day. If you begin to worry when you get into bed, say to yourself, "No. I've taken care of that already." It sounds simple, but it can work if you let it.

The Relaxation Response: Melt Away Stress

People often believe mistakenly that in order to truly relax, they need to take a drink or take a pill. Nothing could be further from the truth. Your body can do the job on its own if you let it. At the Whitaker Wellness Institute we teach a technique called the *relaxation response.* Developed by Dr.

Herbert Benson of the Mind/Body Medical Institute at the New England Deaconess Hospital and the Harvard Medical Institute, the relaxation response can soothe the spirit and help the body wind down after a hectic day.

The relaxation response involves a wide range of physiological changes. Oxygen consumption is decreased, the heart rate slows down, muscles relax, and blood pressure can drop. The best news of all, however, is that the relaxation response is a state of deep relaxation you can elicit yourself in order to rejuvenate your body and freshen your mind. Continual practice of the relaxation response will bring feelings of increased control over the details of your life and the sense that even your body's physiological reactions can be brought under control. Many people who practice the relaxation response experience a greater sense of self-assurance and a decrease in stress-related symptoms, including insomnia.

Here's a quick guide to acquiring the relaxation response based on the technique designed by Dr. Benson:

First a few preliminaries:

- Identify fifteen minutes in your schedule, preferably early in the evening, before dinner, for a regular session. Arrange a time when there will be no distractions.
- Keep a watch or clock within sight so you can check it periodically. You want to commit the full time to this endeavor.

How to elicit the response:

- Choose a focus word or short phrase that has some resonance for you. It could be a word such as "peace" or the beginning of a prayer or saying.
- Sitting quietly in a comfortable position, close your eyes.
- Breathe slowly and normally, repeating the word silently as you exhale.

- Relax your muscles, starting from your head and neck and moving down toward your toes. Consciously sense each body part as you go.
- Keep breathing evenly and repeating your word. If and when other thoughts intrude, do not rush from them but instead gently accept that they exist. Move past them with a kind of "yes-but-later" attitude.
- Do this for about fifteen minutes (checking the clock occasionally), and when you are finished, sit quietly for a few extra minutes with your eyes closed at first and then open.

At the end of this time you will likely feel peaceful and calm, and ready to sleep without the worries of your day haunting you at night.

ARE YOU GETTING ENOUGH EXERCISE?

People who do not exercise on a regular basis are more likely to have sleep problems. A recent Stanford University study of three dozen adults with sleep complaints found that a brisk walk or a low-impact aerobic session every couple of days cut falling asleep time in half and extended sleep by almost an hour.

I personally believe twenty to thirty minutes of daily exercise is the best sleep remedy, and if you are following my workout routine at least three days a week, I bet you are already getting a better night's sleep. The key is that you cannot exercise any old time you want. Exercise should be completed about two to three hours before bedtime because it revs up the body and in turn clears the head and makes you feel alert. It takes your body time to wind down, so don't exercise too late in the evening or you may have difficulty falling asleep.

IS YOUR DIET CONDUCIVE TO SLEEP?

Restless sleep could easily indicate a problem with your diet. In fact, diet is a major cause of insomnia for many people. Certain foods can encourage and/or disturb a good night's sleep. Again, by following my Age Loss Program's food plan, you should already be avoiding foods that disrupt sleep, but consider the following pointers.

1. Forget the warm milk myth. It actually may not be the best choice at bedtime. Although the calcium and L-tryptophan in milk are natural sedatives, dairy products and other fatty foods can be difficult to digest. As a result they keep your body working overtime.

2. Avoid refined carbohydrates. The same age-accelerating carbohydrates that cause sudden increases in blood sugar can interfere with your sleep. Initially they may leave you feeling wired, but the blood sugar drop that follows may wake you in the middle of the night. Sugary desserts and soft drinks close to bedtime (or any time for that matter) will exacerbate this problem.

3. Drink eight glasses of water a day. If you are following Age Loss cuisine, you are already doing this, but here's another good reason to keep it up: Water flushes out the toxins from your body, thereby easing the nighttime demands on your liver and digestive system.

Keep in mind that how you eat, not just what you eat, can also impact on your sleep. You should eat a large breakfast, a moderate lunch, and a light dinner. Be sure that the evening meal contains a small serving of some protein such as fish, chicken, or a non-meat protein such as beans. A healthy but light evening meal will help prevent hunger pangs in the middle of the night. Also, don't eat dinner too late in the evening because your body will be too busy digesting your meal to relax. And of course you must be careful about beverages and foods containing stimulants that can keep you tossing and turning all night.

4. Watch your caffeine intake. A cup or two of coffee in the morning isn't going to harm you, but if sleep is a problem, I would avoid drinking caffeinated beverages anytime after breakfast, especially in the afternoon or evening. Caffeine can linger in your bloodstream for as long as eight hours, so it is no surprise that it can interfere with sleep. Admittedly, some people are more sensitive to caffeine than others. Yet many people are more affected by it than they even realize. Research subjects who say they can drink coffee before bedtime and sleep just as well actually have been shown in a laboratory study to slumber less restfully than they thought. Keep in mind also that other caffeinated substances such as chocolate, cola, and tea can result in a poor-quality rest. So avoid those, too, in the afternoons and evenings.

5. Ax the alcohol. We all know that alcohol can help you fall asleep, but here's the rub: As alcohol is metabolized by the body, it releases a natural stimulant that disrupts sleep during the second half of the night. Chronic alcoholics, for example, suffer from abnormal sleep patterns regardless of their age. Their sleep is usually disrupted by hundreds of awakenings during the night. If you are in the habit of having several drinks each night to help you get some rest, withdraw gradually. Cut down to one drink per night for a few days, then to one very diluted drink. Finally, cut out the alcohol altogether and opt for a glass of diluted fruit juice. I also recommend some natural sleep enhancers that can help you sleep like a baby and won't cause a hangover. (For more information see page 210.)

6. Nix the nicotine. Here's yet another reason not to smoke. Nicotine is a stimulant and therefore can keep you awake. Smokers often have a lot of trouble falling asleep because cigarettes raise blood pressure, speed up the heart rate, and stimulate brain-wave activity. Smokers also tend to wake up more in the middle of the night, possibly because their bodies are experiencing withdrawal symptoms. Obviously, the best thing you can do for yourself is to quit smoking altogether, but if you are not willing or ready, at least try to cut down on the number of cigarettes you have in the evening near bedtime. And when you are unable to sleep, the worst thing you can do is light a cigarette. Pick up a magazine instead.

IS YOUR ENVIRONMENT CONDUCIVE TO SLEEP?

Sometimes the solution to our problems is right under our nose, and we don't even know it. The right sleep environment can make all the difference between a restful night or a fitful one. Everything matters, from the sheets (Madam Chiang Kai-shek, it is said, took her own sheets with her when she traveled—even to the White House) to the sort of clock that rests at your bedside. No detail is too small to ruin your sleep. The list could actually be endless, but here's a sample of what you should think about:

> Are your sheets fresh?
> Is the blanket the right weight?
> Is the bed big enough?
> Do the innersprings of the mattress make too much noise?
> Are the pillows the correct density for you?

In other words, are you comfortable when you get into your bed at night? Here are some other, less obvious things to think about:

Adjust the room temperature. Is your thermostat set to automatically shift at night? Is that temperature *really* comfortable for you? When you get into bed at night, do you find yourself piling on or throwing off covers? Lots of adjusting might mean the room temperature is not good for you and could result in a restless night as you repeatedly wake either too hot or too cold.

Dampen the noise. If noise is keeping you awake, try eliminating as much of it as possible by using carpeting and draperies. Most of us can easily accommodate a relatively steady noise. It's the occasional loud noises such as an airplane or fire engine that cause a problem. If your environment is clamorous, a noise screen such as a sound box can help. A white noise machine (which emits a steady but low-frequency noise) can muffle sounds by producing a soothing neutral tone without a pattern or message. Even running a fan or air conditioner can help.

Turn off the clock. Ticking clocks will not do. Neither will a bright illuminated digital clock. People who can't sleep often fixate on the glowing numerals, thereby increasing their level of frustration as they watch each second and minute go by. If you must keep a clock by the side of your bed, at least tone down the glow; otherwise, put the clock under your bed or in a top dresser drawer so that you can't obsess over the time.

SCHEDULE TIME FOR RELAXATION AND SLEEP

All other factors aside, many people are sleep deprived simply because of their lifestyle. Are your work hours ridiculous? Are you staying up too late watching television? Are you going to bed too keyed up by whatever activity you've been engaged in minutes before? If you find that you are hyperalert when your

208

head hits the pillow, you will not be able to unwind or fall asleep. For the next ten weeks I want you to set aside time each night to wind down, get an evening ritual going, and stick to a schedule.

In other words, you can't just climb into bed and fall asleep immediately without getting yourself into sleep mode hours before. Try to make your evenings as relaxing and restorative as possible. Start winding down after dinner or as early as your schedule allows. Try to do the same relaxing, no-stress activities every night before bed. Select a cue that it's time to settle in. Do your evening skin care regimen (see Step 3). Scan a book (but not one that will keep you up all night), water plants, or flip through a magazine. Try to maintain the same order every night. It will help your body understand that it is time to wind down. Keep in mind that you should never take a hot bath before climbing into bed. The hot bath can actually be stimulating because it heats up your body temperature just at a time when you are cooling down in preparation for sleep. Don't get me wrong—soaking in a hot tub is a great way to relieve tension and escape from everyday life. Just do it at least one hour before bedtime. See below for wonderful herbal baths that will help you relax and unwind.

IS THERE A PHYSICAL PROBLEM?

Finally, there are the physical conditions that can interfere with sleep. Chemical imbalances in the body and medical problems such as sleep apnea (a condition in which you stop breathing temporarily and snore loudly when you try to catch your breath) can be at the root of your problem. If insomnia is a chronic problem, it is a good idea to check with your doctor to rule out an underlying physical cause.

For women, menopause is a time when sleep problems are likely to strike. It is not uncommon for menopausal women to be awakened by a hot flash or to wake up too early. Some of the natural sleep remedies recommended below can help end these problems.

THROW OUT THE SLEEPING PILLS: USE NATURAL SLEEP ENHANCERS

Even if you follow my suggestions and do everything right, some of you may still have difficulty falling asleep. Don't worry, help is available. If you've had sleep problems in the past, it will take more than one or two nights to teach your body new habits. You may be tempted to give up and reach for a sleeping pill. My advice is don't.

Prescription sleeping pills are not the panacea you might like to think they are. They are addictive, and the doses often have to be increased to maintain effectiveness. If you abruptly stop taking them, you may find it even more difficult to fall asleep—a problem known as "rebound insomnia." Sleeping pills also tend to disrupt normal sleep cycles by reducing both dreaming and deep sleep, and may leave you groggy for most of the morning.

Over-the-counter sleep aids are no better. They use sedating antihistamines, which are not as effective as prescription sleeping pills and will also leave you with significant drowsiness in the morning.

If you are looking for some good, safe, natural sleep inducers, turn to supplements and herbs, which have been safe and effective sleeping aids for thousands of years. They are available in many different forms, including teas, capsules, and scented oils. Studies have shown that herbs can act like mild sedatives to relax the nervous system and shorten the time it takes to fall asleep. Herbs are gentler to the system and have few harmful side effects. Here are some herbs you might like to add to your nighttime ritual. You can use them individually or together.

Lavender: This herb has been used for at least one thousand years in various folk remedies for insomnia. Those ancient healers knew what they were doing.

Researchers in England recently tested whether lavender oil could be used as a treatment for insomnia for nursing home residents. Four patients who had been on sleep medication for up to three years had their sleep monitored for six weeks. For the first two weeks the medication was tapered off. The second two weeks, the patients were given no medication. The last two weeks, the patients did not get any medication but their rooms were perfumed with lavender oil. Researchers found that the patients had difficulty sleeping during the second two weeks when their medication was discontinued, but amazingly, during the last two weeks they slept equally as well with the lavender oil as they did with their medication. In other words, the lavender oil worked as well as a sleeping pill! Of course, the advantages of lavender oil are that it does not have to be ingested, it is nonaddicting, and there are no side effects.

A number of lavender sleep products are available in herb shops and health food stores. Recently, I tried a lavender-scented eye pillow that I found in my local herb shop. You simply place it over your eyes at bedtime. The scent of the lavender is incredibly relaxing, and before you know it, you're fast asleep.

Chamomile: This herb is well known for its relaxing effects. Drink a warm cup of chamomile tea or take a warm bath with lavender oil an hour or two before sleep time. As an alternative you might want to try adding a quart of strong chamomile tea to your bathwater for a truly relaxing pre-sleep ablution. (Chamomile is a member of the daisy family, which includes ragweed. Anyone who is allergic to ragweed should avoid chamomile.)

Passion flower: This herb has several powerful and interesting constituents, and it was used by the Aztecs as both a sedative and an analgesic. Passion flower is available in capsules. Take two capsules at bedtime on those nights that you need help sleeping.

Valerian: This is the most druglike of the herbs. It can be as effective in small doses as barbiturates in reducing the time it takes to fall asleep, but unlike drugs, valerian actually reduces morning sleepiness. Although the usual dose is two capsules before bedtime, valerian can be unpredictable because it overstimulates some people rather than sedates them. If you have never taken it before, start with one capsule to see how it will affect you. If you find that it revs you up rather than calms you down, don't use it.

Herbal mixture: Several herbal sleep aid products contain combinations of passion flower, valerian, chamomile, and other herbs that have a calming effect on the body. They are sold in health food stores and are remarkably effective.

TRY MELATONIN

If my herbal remedies don't do the trick, add melatonin to your sleep regimen.

Because it has been in the news so much recently, people often ask me about melatonin. I take melatonin myself every night, and I recommend it to my patients, especially those with sleep problems. Melatonin is a natural hormone known for its ability to regulate sleep cycles, and for many people it is a veritable cure for insomnia. Produced in the pineal gland, a pea-sized structure embedded deep in the brain, it controls the body's circadian rhythm, which informs us when it's time to sleep and awaken. Melatonin is also a potent antioxidant and has been shown in animal studies to significantly extend life and reverse many of the telltale signs of aging.

Melatonin is at its peak level in childhood, drops during adolescence when other hormones kick in, and continues to decrease as you age. By sixty our pineal gland is producing half the amount of melatonin it did when we were twenty. Some researchers believe that the decline in melatonin is responsible for age-related sleep disorders and many symptoms associated with aging.

Taking tiny doses of melatonin supplements at nighttime can shorten the amount of time it takes to fall asleep and restore normal sleep cycles. Unlike sleeping pills, melatonin is nonaddictive and does not interfere with the amount or quality of REM and Delta sleep. Melatonin is sold in tablet and capsules at health food stores and pharmacies, and should be taken only before bedtime.

How much should you take? That all depends. Some people are extraordinarily sensitive to melatonin and become very sleepy after taking only 1 milligram. Others find that they need to take 5 or 6 milligrams a night; in rare cases, some people find that it has no effect whatsoever. You will have to experiment to see what works for you. If you have difficulty falling asleep, try .5 to 2 milligrams of melatonin about half an hour before bedtime. Most people will sleep soundly using 1 to 2 milligrams. But if that doesn't do the trick, try another 1 to 2 milligrams. If you still aren't sleepy, try another 2 milligrams, but I wouldn't recommend any more than that. If six milligrams does not affect you, then you are probably one of those rare people who are not affected by melatonin.

Some people should absolutely not take melatonin. I do not recommend melatonin on a regular basis to those under forty. In addition, melatonin should not be combined with tranquilizers. And since melatonin stimulates immune function, it may not be safe for people with overactive immune systems, such as those with rheumatoid arthritis or lupus.

A sleep problem itself can be very stressful. The moment you place your head on the pillow, you might find yourself riddled with sleep anxieties: "What if I toss and turn for hours? I'm so tired! I have to be fresh tomorrow. I can't stand this anymore." Pretty soon you are up all night from the sheer panic of not sleeping. The same thing is likely to happen if you wake up in the middle of the night and can't fall back to sleep.

Some of the suggestions in this chapter will work immediately, others may take longer. Obviously, it will take a few days or weeks to establish a pattern that your body responds to. You may still have some restless nights until you have retrained your body to sleep, but by the end of ten weeks you should be sleeping better and reaping the benefits. Here are some final tips and suggestions to help you sleep on those nights that you just can't seem to:

- If you can't sleep, *don't* stay in bed watching TV, paying bills, or chatting on the phone. You want your bed to be a cue to sleep.
- Don't toss and turn, trying to will yourself back to sleep. Get out of bed as soon as you feel frustrated, and go into another room. Do something relaxing that you enjoy. Read a dull book or listen to soothing music. Return to bed as soon as you feel sleepy. If you still can't fall off to sleep, get up again. Repeat until you do fall asleep.
- Don't obsess about not sleeping. Tell yourself if it happens again tomorrow night, that won't be terrible, either. You can handle tomorrow even if you're tired.

- Don't nap during the day. If you have difficulty falling asleep, save sleep for the night, or you may not be tired enough to sleep.
- Don't hit the snooze button. Get out of bed when you open your eyes in the morning. Falling in and out of sleep will interfere with your biological clock.
- Go to bed later and wake up earlier. If you have more than occasional insomnia and it takes you hours to fall asleep, try going to bed an hour later every night and setting the alarm a little earlier. The process will keep you out of bed when you can't sleep and will help get you into a sleep/wake cycle that works for YOU.

Everyone needs a good night's sleep. I can't stress this often enough. A good night's sleep varies for everyone, but basically your sleep should be continuous and uninterrupted in any significant way. It should not be hard to fall asleep or difficult to wake up. This is critical to your emotional and physical health. Drugs will not give you the kind of natural and restful slumber you need, but now you know that there is a lot more you can do to acquire a good rest. It is essential to sleep well consistently in order to recapture a more youthful and healthful way of life.

Step 8

RECHARGE THE SPIRIT

Enhance your feelings of joy and well-being
Shed the stress to shed the years
Awaken your senses and relax your body and mind

THE FIRST STEP TO recharging the spirit is to reduce the negative impact of stress on our lives; it can drain us of our vitality and energy. Although it is impossible to eliminate stress completely, it is well within our power to develop better coping mechanisms so that stressful situations do not exact as steep a toll.

JUST SAY NO . . . AT LEAST FOR TEN WEEKS

One of the leading causes of stress is having too much to do and being pulled in too many different directions. I urge you to lighten your load as much as possible for the next ten weeks and carve out some personal time. Take out your calendar. Look over your commitments. Are they all absolutely necessary? Is there anything that can be postponed or even eliminated? Can you delegate some of your jobs to others? I'm not telling you to turn your life upside down or to ignore your responsibilities. All I am suggesting is that you save fifteen minutes a day for yourself.

FIND AN OUTLET FOR STRESS

Though stress is an inevitable part of daily life, "stressed out" doesn't have to be. We all need an outlet for stress. If we can't vent our emotions in a healthy way, we may completely deplete ourselves by turning all that negative energy inward. This results in physical symptoms such as stomachaches, headaches, and even heart palpitations. Clearly, we need to manage and modulate our emotional and physical reactions through *positive* action. If you're having a tough day at home with the kids or if a coworker angers you, don't just sit back and simmer. When you feel anxious and keyed up, acknowledge that you're under stress and then *do something to alleviate it.*

One of the best things to do when you are revved up is to move your body. Exercise helps deplete the stress hormones that are circulating through your body so that you can calm down faster. Even if you don't have the time or inclination for a full workout, a brisk five- or ten-minute walk will release tension and help you unwind.

If you don't want to release tension through exercise, listening to music is another instant cure for stress. Whether you are at home or at the office, find a quiet place to sit down, slip on some headphones, and spend ten minutes listening to a favorite cassette or CD. Even something as simple as keeping a "stress ball" at your desk that you can squeeze when you are angry may be just the outlet you need to keep stress under control.

Another simple way of eliminating stress is to stop and smell the flowers. It's easy to become consumed by what's wrong or by what we don't have and then overlook the pleasures we do enjoy in life. The sense that we are completely "without" can evoke a tremendous stress response. If you want to start coping more effectively in the down time, it is critical that you take some time during the day to remind yourself of what is good. If it helps, make a list of your blessings so that every time you find yourself focusing solely on the negative, you can balance it with the positive things in your life.

RELAXATION TECHNIQUES

In much the same way that physical exercise helps us build muscle, mental exercises and relaxation help us alleviate stress and strengthen our psyche. Here are some simple solutions to alleviating stress and lifting your spirit. Choose the one that works best for you, or better yet, incorporate them all into your ten-week Age Loss Program.

Meditation

Meditation is an ancient technique that will help you find that place in your mind which is a sanctuary from the "noise" of daily living.

Often a component of Yoga, it is the part of your spiritual and emotional self that is the essential you. It's a quiet place, and when you get there, those worries and concerns that are dragging you down will simply be elsewhere. When you are finished meditating, you will be better able to put things in perspective.

To truly plumb the spiritual aspect of the meditative experience, it would be wise to seek the help of a qualified teacher. But for now I will show you a largely physiological technique that taps into the mind/body connection and helps you arrive at the silent place where your body and mind can enjoy a deep peace.

Not unlike the relaxation response described in Step 7, this technique involves sitting in a quiet place with no distractions. It, too, encourages the gentle turning away of intrusive negative thoughts and a journey inward during which you experience your body in a new way. The key is that the meditative technique centers on breathing.

1. Sitting quietly with your hands in your lap or gently resting beside you, close your eyes and breathe lightly and normally.
2. Listen as the air is passed down into your lungs through your nostrils and then softly up and out. The breath should be gentle and easy. As your breathing relaxes try making it a little lighter. If you begin to feel short of breath, breathe in a bit.
3. Allow your body to dictate what you need listening as fully as you can, concentrating on the internal sounds and sensations of air moving in, through, and out of your body. Do this for ten to twenty minutes.

By paying attention to your breathing, you will sink deeper and deeper into a state of relaxation, thus quieting your mind. You will feel calm and yet refreshed, and ready to face the rest of your day.

Aromatherapy

Sometimes the answer to stress may be right under your nose —literally. Growing in popularity by leaps and bounds, aromatherapy utilizes the power of scent to soothe, relax, and heal. Nearly two thousand years ago, Hippocrates, the father of modern medicine, noted that "the way to health is to have an aromatic bath and a scented massage every day." Since ancient times, healers have used the essential oils from spices and herbs to treat various illnesses of the body and the mind. Today, essential oils are sold in thousands of shops around the country, including herb shops (such as The Body Shop and Aveeda), health food stores, and even department stores. There are dozens of oils to choose from, and generally you can use one oil at a time or combine several. Most herb shops will let you sample several oils so that you can custom design your own aromatherapy treatment. Remember, a little oil goes a long way; you only need to use a few drops to experience the full benefit of aromatherapy.

Studies have documented the power of essential oils to relax and recharge the body and mind. They can be used in various ways and should never be ingested. Choose the method or methods that you like best. Once inhaled through the nose, essential oils stimulate the olfactory organs, which are linked to the areas of the brain that control emotions. When rubbed on the skin, essential oils stimulate a reaction in the nerve endings on the skin's surface, which can trigger an emotional response.

Here are the most effective and popular methods.

Inhale it. Do not inhale an essential oil directly from the bottle because the scent may be too strong and could be irritating. Instead, boil one quart of water and add ten drops of oil. Inhale the steam.

Scent the room. Another way to safely get the benefit of essential oils is to put a few drops of oil in a special lamp called an aroma defuser. It heats the oil and dispenses the scent throughout the room. There are numerous lamps on the market; some particularly attractive ones are the Pangaea lamp and lamps by Aromaland sold at bath and body stores.

Bathe in it. Add five to ten drops of essential oil to a warm bath. Relax in the tub for at least fifteen minutes.

Apply it to your skin. Diluted essential oils designed specifically for external use can be used directly on the skin. (Do not, however, use a full-strength oil on the skin; it will be too irritating.) Rub five drops of diluted oil on your neck, chest, and wrists. Reapply every four or five hours, or when you feel low.

There are dozens of essential oils, and each elicits different emotional responses. Here is a list of oils that are particularly good for reinvigorating the body and the mind.

Roman Chamomile	When you are tense or irritable, chamomile oil can soothe the spirit. Keep a bottle of chamomile oil in your desk at work!
Citrus	Citrus oil (particularly grapefruit and orange) will lift you out of the blues. In one Japanese study, after using citrus aromatherapy for four to eleven weeks, patients who had been taking antidepressants daily were able to cut back or even eliminate their medication.
Bergamot	This oil will uplift the spirit and put you in a good mood.
Geranium	This oil will help control mood swings.
Rosemary	This oil has a stimulating effect on the body and mind and is reputed to improve memory.

Aromatherapy is a wonderful way to unwind and quickly recharge your spirit.

Light Up Your Life

Something as simple and basic as light can profoundly affect your mood. I don't know anyone whose spirit isn't lifted on a bright, sunny spring day, and who doesn't feel just a bit down on a dark and gloomy winter day? There is a physiological basis for these shifts in mood. Our brains are wired to react to different types of light, and exposure to light and dark controls the body's internal time clock, or circadian rhythm. When light enters the eye, it stimulates the production of hormones in the brain that regulate virtually every bodily activity, from sleep to body temperature to sexual function to even mood. Not surprisingly, light deprivation can cause physical and psychological problems. For some, these problems are more severe and signal a condition known as Seasonal Affective Disorder (SAD), which strikes during winter months when the days are the shortest. For most of us, however, light has a more subtle yet very real effect on our mood.

One problem is that most of us do not spend enough time basking in the right kind of light. The sun emits full-spectrum light, which means that it contains all wavelengths of color. Full-spectrum light is necessary to trigger the impulses within the brain that control important bodily functions.

Artificial indoor light, which is usually fluorescent or in-candescent, is not full spectrum and therefore does not have the same uplifting effect. Quite the contrary, in some people it has a depressing effect. Since we spend most of our time indoors, we are exposed primarily to artificial light. There are some simple things you can do, however, to let more of the right kind of light in your life—at least over the next ten weeks.

LET THE SUN SHINE IN.
This is as simple as it gets: Pull up the shades, open the dra-peries, and let the light in. Sunlight will stimulate your brain and give you a natural lift. This is a safe way to take advantage of sunlight without exposing your skin to ultraviolet rays.

SWITCH TO FULL-SPECTRUM LIGHTS.
Put full-spectrum lights in one or two of the rooms at home or at work where you spend the most time. You don't have to

buy new fixtures. Full-spectrum tubes for preexisting fluorescent fixtures and full-spectrum bulbs for lamps and chan-
deliers are sold in lighting stores and by catalog. (See the
Resources section for more information.) I have used full-
spectrum lights in my office for almost twenty years, and
when I leave my office with its crisp energizing bluish lights
and walk into other office buildings with yellowish, polluted
light, I can actually *feel* the difference.

GO EASY ON THE SUNGLASSES.
Colored glasses grossly distort the light energy entering our
brains. Environmental Lighting Concepts has a line of tinted
sunglasses that reduce the intensity of light but allow the full
spectrum to penetrate the eyes.

DON'T HIBERNATE.
Especially during the winter try to plan a brief walk out in the
sunshine. Dress warmly and let the rays lift you out of the
"winter blues."

The most important thing to keep in mind is that not all
light is the same. Recognize the kind you need and make sure
you expose yourself to it whenever possible. A few minutes
with full-spectrum light can keep sagging spirits from deepening and turn a decent mood into a spirited one.

When Simple Solutions Don't Work: Try Kava

There are many natural supplements that can reduce anxiety
and boost your spirits, which are all sold over the counter at
health food stores and pharmacies. If the simple techniques
that I have already described don't work for you, you may
want to try Kava, a wonderful, soothing supplement that is
particularly good for people who are under a great deal of
stress.

If you are feeling stressed out or anxious, I recommend that you include the following supplement in your daily plan for at least the ten weeks that you are on the Age Loss Program, if not longer.

For thousands of years the herb kava has been used in the South Seas as a mood enhancer and treatment for anxiety. Today, kava is growing in popularity in the West, and kava teas and capsules are sold in health food stores and pharmacies.

Kava contains biologically active compounds called kavalactones that have been shown to be effective against stress, anxiety, and muscle tension. Unlike tranquilizers, kava will not leave you feeling groggy or "drugged"; instead, it promotes a feeling of tranquillity and well-being. Even better, kava is nonaddictive.

The kavalactones in kava have a profoundly positive effect on the region of the brain that controls emotion. There have been more than eight hundred studies of the benefits of kava as an anti-anxiety agent in Europe, and most of them have verified that kava works as well as, if not better than, many prescription anti-anxiety drugs.

Kava is also an important part of the social life of South Sea residents. The kava ceremony, which involves drinking a strong kava drink, is reserved for honored guests. Dignitaries who have visited the South Seas—from Pope John Paul II to Hillary Clinton—have participated in the kava ceremony. What a nice way to relax your guests and make them feel at home!

If you feel anxious and stressed out, I recommend that you take 60 milligrams of kava daily. Like many other herbs, kava has a cumulative effect, which means that it will take about four weeks to notice an improvement in anxiety. You should feel better long before you have completed the Age Loss Program, and if kava works well for you, you may want to continue on it for as long as you need it. (If you are currently taking a prescription drug for anxiety, work with your doctor to wean yourself off it slowly and to start kava.)

Get Involved

Perhaps the most important technique to reduce stress is also the most basic: People need to feel connected to the world at large.

There is a great deal of evidence linking social support with physical well-being. The research indicates that having a significant number of close social relationships is associated with a longer and healthier life.

A study conducted by David Spiegel, M.D., the director of the Psychosocial Treatment Lab at Stanford University School of Medicine, looked at a group of women suffering from comparable breast cancer and receiving comparable medical care. He followed those who were in support groups and those who were not. The women who were part of the support groups lived an average of eighteen months longer.

James House of the University of Michigan gathered data on the social patterns of 2,754 adults interviewed during visits to their doctor. House found that the most socially active men were three times less likely to die within nine to twelve years than those of a similar age who were most isolated.

James Goodwin at the Medical College of Wisconsin and his colleagues conducted a study on cancer survival in several thousand patients and found the married cancer patients did better and lived longer than the unmarried.

A review article of the research on social interaction and health published in the journal *Science* noted that the relationship between social isolation and early death is as statistically strong as the relationship between dying and smoking!

There are, of course, many theories as to why social relationships may be linked to physical health. It could be that when people feel others care about them, they actually take better care of themselves. They might be more likely to avoid bad habits such as smoking, drug use, and excessive drinking, substances that can weaken their cardiovascular, immune, and nervous systems.

Still, some researchers looking beyond these behavioral explanations have done studies that suggest the connection with others has direct physical benefits. The "stress hormones" that pump into the bloodstream during difficult times —which can lead to an elevated heart rate, poor metabolism, and depression—may be dramatically inhibited by the support of others.

Seymour Levine, a psychologist at Stanford University, conducted an experiment in which a squirrel monkey was given a mild shock whenever a light flashed. Eventually he discontinued the shock, but every time the light was flashed, the monkey continued to have a stress reaction in which its blood levels of stress hormone rose. However, if another monkey was placed in the cage with him for company and the light flashed, the stressed monkey produced only half the amount of stress hormone. When five other monkeys were placed in the cage, there was no increase. The existence of friends, it would seem, may shield our physical selves from the consequences of stress.

Having a sense of connection to the world is essential for our mental health. Whether it be getting involved in a community activity, going to your local church or temple, or just maintaining your friendships, nurturing the spirit is an important part of staying healthy and whole. Do something special to send your spirits soaring over the next ten weeks. Whether it's meditation, aromatherapy, or taking a few minutes out of your day to practice relaxation, set aside the time to care for your psyche in a way that is meaningful to you. I believe that happiness and joy, like good nutrition, strengthens the body, soothes the mind, and has a rejuvenating effect on both.

Step 9

⟋

REINVIGORATE YOUR IMMUNE SYSTEM

Restore your body's natural healing power
Build up your resistance to infection
Bounce back faster from colds, flu,
and other common ailments

REMEMBER WHEN YOU COULD shake off a cold practically over-night instead of suffering through lingering sniffles and aches for a week or two? Remember when a bout of flu came and went in a matter of days and didn't leave you out of commission for weeks at a time? Remember when a cough was just a cough and didn't mushroom into a full-blown respiratory infection that dogged you all winter long? And serious ill-nesses? I'll bet you never even gave them a second thought when you were younger.

Once you hit your 40s or 50s, however, things began to change. You got sick more often, and you didn't bounce back as easily as you used to. And you began to worry more about serious illnesses, such as cancer.

What's happened? The answer is that your immune system is showing signs of the midlife energy crises. The same destructive forces that are accelerating the aging process everywhere else in your body are also wearing down your immune system, your natural bodyguard.

Your immune system is a cellular fortress that stands between you and disease. Your immune system protects you against bacteria, viruses, environmental toxins, and cancer-causing agents. Although the weakening of our immune system is not as visible as the graying of our hair or the wrinkling of our skin, it is a sign that the aging process is taking hold. Forget the old saw, "You're only as old as you feel," and substitute "You're only as young as your immune system," because the younger your immune system, the younger you will be . . . and feel.

How do we keep our immune system young? The answer is found in the same Age Loss Program's rule that you've heard before: Inaction accelerates aging. You can have a strong, youthful, resilient immune system for your entire life, provided you take the right steps to preserve it. My method of boosting immune function will do just that.

YOUR IMMUNE SYSTEM: THE ARMY WITHIN

First, let me tell you a little about your immune system, which is probably the most complex of all our body systems. Only within the past few decades have scientists begun to understand how it works because it has been hard to put a finger on precisely what the immune system is. Unlike your circulatory, nervous, and digestive systems, which are composed of specific and identifiable body parts, your immune system is nebulous and diffuse. It is composed of hundreds of different types of cells scattered throughout the body, each having remarkably specific functions.

The primary role of the immune system is to keep you out of harm's way and protect your body from numerous foreign invaders. We humans share the earth with billions of microorganisms—bacteria, viruses, fungi, protozoa, and parasites—all of them looking for a foothold in our bodies. At the same time that the immune system is fending off our foes, however, it must be very careful not to attack our own body tissue. Autoimmune diseases, such as rheumatoid arthritis and lupus, occur when immune cells can no longer distinguish between friend and foe, and turn their full force on the body's own tissues and organs.

When we are under attack from microorganisms, our immune system rallies to our defense in several important ways. Each immune cell has its own particular job. I like to think of "B cells" as the bouncers of the body because they "throw out" uninvited guests. When a foreign substance enters the body, B cells quickly produce antibodies that attack and try to destroy it. Antibodies have good memories, and when the body encounters an infection it has "met" before, the antibodies are already prepared for the challenge. This is how we develop immunity against certain infections. For example, most people get chicken pox only once in their lives because with the first exposure their bodies develop antibodies that repel it on sight in the future.

The Avenging T Cells

If a virus or bacteria should get past the B cells, it will encounter an army of several different types of angry T cells. Some T cells engage in "hand-to-hand" combat with unwelcome invaders, and they are critical for our survival. Others known as "suppressor cells" do not attack foreign invaders but prevent other T cells from attacking the host—that's *you*. Another group of immune cells called natural killer cells seek out and identify cells in your body that reproduce abnormally, including cancer cells, and kill them. You have undoubtedly heard a great deal about T cells in recent years in the context of AIDS and the HIV virus. What makes AIDS so insidious is that the virus that causes it knocks out T cells, leaving the body defenseless against other infections.

Our immune system is an incredible ally, but we experience a dramatic decline in immune function as we age. We call this decline *immunosenescence.* Our B cells become sloppy and don't produce antibodies as efficiently. Our disease-fighting T cells become less effective, which is why it becomes harder to shake off an infection. Suppressor T cells can no longer distinguish friend from foe and often attack the body's own tissue, causing the incidence of autoimmune diseases to rise dramatically with age. And our natural killer cells become lazy and let abnormal cells proliferate, with the result that the rate of cancer rises exponentially with age.

My patient Janet is typical of the numerous patients I see who are suffering the effects of immunosenescence. From the time she was in her late twenties, Janet worked long hours in a family-owned business. At the same time she raised three children, was active in the PTA, and served as a volunteer at her church. She rarely missed a day at work; as she put it, "I was too busy to get sick."

When Janet reached her mid-forties, however, things changed. She started getting frequent colds and coughs, some of which actually required bed rest—unheard of for her. She found, much to her consternation, that she had to cut back on a few activities because she just couldn't keep her old pace. Now she is forty-nine, and for the last year and a half has been battling an unshakable upper respiratory condition. Her family physician has given a series of antibiotics, each one stronger than the last; each one seemed to help for a while, but then the symptoms returned.

Day in and day out I see patients such as Janet, people in their forties, fifties, and older who are sick and tired of being sick and tired. They complain that they are felled by every cold or flu bug that comes along and that they go down harder and stay down longer. All of this is happening because their immune systems aren't functioning at full capacity.

My approach to treating these patients, who comprise a significant percentage of my practice, is startlingly simple. If they are already sick, like Janet, I make them well again by reinvigorating their immune system so it can overcome the infection. If they are not sick, my goal is to reinvigorate their immune system to prevent infection from taking hold.

Once Janet began my method of reinvigorating her immune system, her life turned around. No longer is she defeated by every infection she encounters, and if she does catch a cold, it is gone in a matter of days. It's as if she has turned the clock back a full ten years!

If necessary, I of course prescribe an antibiotic to eliminate a bacterial infection, but I do not rely solely or heavily on antibiotics. I believe the job of medicine is not to kill off foreign invaders but to strengthen the immune system so that the body can fight its own fights, as it is meant to. My goal is to help my patients achieve an optimal level of *wellness* through specific lifestyle changes and nutritional measures that reinvigorate their immune systems.

My wellness approach is the foundation of the Whitaker Wellness Institute, but the concept did not originate with me. In ancient China wealthy families employed physicians to keep them well. If a member of the family became ill, this meant that the doctor wasn't doing his job, and so the doctor was not entitled to get paid! (Just imagine how different Western medicine would be if we adopted this concept!)

Steps 1 through 8 of the ten-week Age Loss Program will contribute to strengthening your immunity, and many of you will not need to do anything else. If you feel that you need to give your immune system an additional boost, however, I am now going to offer ways that you can do so over the next ten weeks.

STRENGTHENING YOUR IMMUNE SYSTEM FROM WITHIN

Take the probiotic approach. "Probiotic" is a general term for microorganisms that do not kill bacteria and other unwanted invaders directly but bolster the body's own defenses against disease. Many probiotics are themselves bacteria that live in the intestines and play a role in digestion. Unlike disease-carrying bacteria, these "friendly" bacteria work in tandem with our immune system to keep us healthy. As we age, we experience a drop in "good bacteria" and an increase in intestinal pathogens. It is therefore imperative to maintain youthful levels of probiotics, and to do so I recommend probiotic supplements on page 235. But it's important that you understand how they work with your body.

Your intestines are home to 100 *trillion* microscopic organisms, including one hundred to four hundred different species of bacteria. These organisms outnumber the cells of the body! Interestingly, your body does not go to war with them; it is as if, through evolution, they've become a part of you.

The most beneficial of the friendly bacteria are bifidobacterium, lactobacillus acidophilus, and lactobacillus bulgaricus. Think of them as good bacteria, because in addition to playing an integral role in the digestive and absorption processes, they perform many other vital functions. One of the most important is that they protect us from overgrowth and infection from their not so nice cousins, certain fungi and yeasts with which they share space. Fungi and yeasts produce toxic and carcinogenic substances that cause digestive problems and may injure the intestines. If left unchecked, they may be absorbed into the bloodstream and contribute to other diseases. The most exciting research on good bacteria is their role in supporting the immune system. Bifidobacteria, in particular, have inhibitory effects on "bad" pathogens, such as salmonella (which causes food poisoning), staphylococcus aureus (which causes staph infections), and candida albicans (which causes yeast infections). Studies have shown that bifidiobacteria have anticarcinogenic and tumor-suppression effects.

One of the reasons I don't like to prescribe antibiotics is that they cannot distinguish between good and bad bacteria. Antibiotics wipe out everything in their path. Even one course of antibiotics can completely alter the makeup of your intestinal flora, killing the good bacteria and allowing the pathogens to proliferate.

Even if you don't take antibiotics, you probably consume them in meat and dairy products. Over 35 million pounds of antibiotics are produced in the United States each year, and livestock get the vast bulk of them. That is why I recommend using only organic, antibiotic-free dairy and poultry products. We promote these good bacteria primarily through food and probiotic supplements:

Immune-friendly food If you are following Age Loss cuisine, you are already eating a diet that is high in fiber-rich complex carbohydrates and therefore very probiotic. Intestinal bacteria "eat" dietary fiber and metabolize it into organic acids that inhibit the growth of bad bacteria. By comparison, a meat-based diet has the opposite effect: It encourages their proliferation. That is precisely why I encourage you to give up red meat at least for the next ten weeks. The Age Loss Program's food plan also includes nonfat or low-fat yogurt, another immune-boosting food that is a rich source of friendly bacteria. According to a study performed at the University of California, people who eat two cartons of yogurt a day have higher blood levels of gamma-interferon, a substance that helps the body ward off infection. Make sure that the yogurt you eat states on the label "made with live and active cultures."

Probiotic supplements If you feel that your immune system needs an additional boost, I recommend that for the next ten weeks you take a daily probiotic supplement, which is sold at health food stores. A probiotic supplement will assure that you retain optimum levels of friendly bacteria so that your immune system retains the youthful advantage. Probiotics are also helpful in overcoming yeast, fungal, and bacterial infections. They come in capsule, liquid, and powder forms, and are easy to take. They have recently become so popular that some of the larger health food stores have an entire probiotic section. There are many brands to choose from, but I recommend Intestinal Care by Ethical Nutrients, Healthy Trinity by Natron, and Kyo-dophilus by America.

If you are ever required to use an antibiotic, it is especially important to take probiotic supplements while you are taking the antibiotic and for up to a month afterward. The supplements will help replace the healthy bacteria that the antibiotics killed along with the bad bacteria.

STRENGTHENING YOUR IMMUNE SYSTEM FROM OUTSIDE

High-Performance Hygiene

An innovative program for strengthening your immune system from the outside in is called the High-Performance Hygiene System. It was developed by Dr. Kenneth Seaton, a remarkable Australian research scientist specializing in aging and immune function. High-performance hygiene is a wonderful tool to rejuvenate your immune system, and I urge you to use it for the ten weeks that you are on the Age Loss Program, particularly if you are vulnerable to infection. Let me tell you why I am so enthusiastic about this innovative method of hygiene.

We've understood for many years that infection is caused by germs. We've also known that proper hygiene can help prevent the spread of infection. What is less well understood is how pathogens gain entry into our bodies and why normal hygiene doesn't protect us against these troublemakers.

Let me ask you a simple question. How do you think you catch a cold? If you're like most folks, you would probably say that you catch a cold from someone else who already has a cold. Well, that's only half the story. In order to catch a cold, you not only have to come into physical contact with a cold virus, but that virus also has to find a port of entry into your body. The possible routes include the mouth, eyes, and nasal passages. You roll out the welcome wagon for cold viruses every time you rub your eyes, chew on a nail, or touch your nose. Washing your hands with soap and water kills some of these viruses but not all of them. Many viruses become embedded in your skin, particularly in your nails or under the cuticles, out of reach of soap and water.

Dr. Seaton's High-Performance Hygiene System includes a special soap that reaches those hard-to-reach viruses. You simply dig your fingernails into his special soap, which is the consistency of soft margarine, and lather up. Rinse your hands, dry them with a clean paper towel, and throw it out. (Do not reuse your hand towel; it is a hotbed of bacteria!) This soap is not medicated or scented, and it is not intended to kill bacteria or viruses. It is designed to emulsify these pathogens so that they're washed away, and it is extremely effective at reducing the pathogen count under the fingernails.

Dr. Seaton also has developed a facial dip for the eyes and nose. You fill a basin with warm water, add his special solution, and dip your face in the water briefly. It's extremely refreshing, and it washes thousands of bacteria and other potential antigens away from the mucous membranes of the eyes and nose. It is also very useful at reducing the effects of exposure to pollen and other allergens. Dr. Seaton recommends that you use the facial dip once in the morning and once at night.

I have prescribed the High-Performance Hygiene System for some of my patients who have chronic respiratory infections, colds, or allergies, and they have experienced excellent results. They find that they get fewer colds, and many find that their allergic symptoms disappear. And the High-Performance Hygiene system appears to do more than just reduce the frequency of colds: It strengthens our immune system by raising levels of albumin, one of the body's most powerful antioxidants. Each time we are exposed to a virus or bacteria, our immune system goes into action by producing antibodies in our bloodstream,where they circulate until the invader is repelled. These antibodies, collectively called immunoglobulins, are one of two main types of protein in your blood. The other is albumin.

Albumin is involved in at least sixty-five different biological functions. It is our body's main transport system, carrying vitamins, minerals, hormones, fatty acids, and other essential substances to their destinations. It is also one of our body's most powerful—and by far its most voluminous—antioxidants. Given the fact that albumin is involved in so many essential functions, it is not surprising that there is a well-established correlation between low albumin levels and mortality. A large number of studies have identified low albumin levels as the most consistent marker for imminent death. The British Heart Study, published in the British medical journal

The Lancet in 1989, followed 7,735 middle-aged British men for 9.2 years. It found that men with the lowest albumin levels had the *highest* rates of death from many different causes.

With a link this strong, researchers have been working on increasing albumin for several decades. Unfortunately, they've mostly struck out, except for Dr. Seaton who spent years tracking albumin and noticed that whenever we get sick, our immunoglobulin levels rise and our albumin levels drop. This happens because they are competing for space in the bloodstream. When antibody levels rise, your body reduces its production of albumin. Even if you don't get sick, your immune system pumps out antibodies that crowd out albumin.

Dr. Seaton reasoned that the only way to lower immunoglobulins in the blood and thus raise albumin is to reduce the viral and bacterial load entering the body. Subsequent studies bore out his theory: Careful washing with his high-performance hygiene products not only lessened the frequency of infections and lowered immunoglobulin levels but also raised albumin. People who used both his hand soap and facial dip had a significant increase in their albumin levels. In sum, high-tech hygiene increases albumin levels by giving your immune system a much-needed rest.

I highly recommend the High-Performance Hygiene System, which is available by mail and includes a book on infectious disease and albumin, four tubs of soap, and four bottles of facial dip. See the Resources section at the end of this book for more information.

Keep Taking the Age Loss ODAs

I already told you about my Age Loss ODAs in Step 1, but I want to stress again the immediate and dramatic effect they have on your immune system.

The power of vitamins and minerals to restore immune

function has been well documented in literally hundreds of studies. Most of these studies show how a particular vitamin or mineral can stimulate antibody production, increase the level of T cells, or rev up natural killer cells. These findings are important and interesting, but I want to tell you about a study that really brings home the message in a meaningful way. Recently, the British medical journal *The Lancet* reported that men and women aged sixty-five who took a daily vitamin and mineral supplement had *half* the number of sick days. To me, the promotion of wellness is the most compelling reason of all to take supplements.

AGE SAVER: Sugar Zaps Immune Cells

Avoid refined sugar: It can depress immune function. Refined sugar has been shown to decrease the activity of immune cells for up to *five hours* after it hits the bloodstream. If you eat a diet high in refined sugar, you are increasing your vulnerability to disease. On the other hand, if you follow the Age Loss Program's food plan, you will be eating the rejuvenating carbohydrates that keep your blood sugar within healthy levels.

For Added Support, Try This High-Tech Supplement

If your immune function is particularly weak—that is, if your sick days still seem to outnumber your well days and you seem to go from infection to infection—you may need to give your immune system an extra boost. I recommend a new high-tech supplement designed to stimulate the thymus gland, the home of the all-important T cells. The thymus, a small gland located behind your breastbone just above your heart, plays a critical part in the immune system. Your army of disease-fighting T cells are born in your blood marrow but migrate to your thymus where they are programmed to differentiate between the cells of the body and foreign proteins.

The decline in immune function that occurs as we age is directly related to a winding down of the thymus gland. The thymus grows rapidly in early childhood, peaks in size and mass at puberty and then begins a gradual downsizing that continues as we age. In many people the thymus gland is barely discernible by age forty. As thymic function decreases, the ability to program T cells is lost, and immune function is compromised.

How do you teach "old" T cells new tricks? Researcher Terry Beardsley, Ph.D., devised a brilliant answer. Dr. Beardsley has isolated a single protein, thymic protein, that may be one of the most powerful immune system stimulants ever discovered. This protein, which is cloned from calf thymus cells, stimulates the immune system by programming T cells, increasing both their numbers and activity. This protein, identical to human protein, has been shown to increase levels of helper T cells, suppressor T cells, natural killer cells, and red and white blood cells. Moreover, it decreased the viral load. It is now being studied as a treatment for numerous diseases, including cancer, AIDS, hepatitis-C, and herpes.

I personally have experienced its power to stimulate immune function. I rarely get sick, but last winter I came down with a severe case of the flu. I was in bed for three days and felt worse than I ever had before. One of my associates brought me some thymic protein, and I took four doses of it during that night. The next morning I was well! Of course, the flu could simply have run its natural course, but the results were so fast and dramatic that no one will convince me that the thymic protein had no effect.

I recommend Biopro Thymic Protein A, which comes in 4-microgram packets, each containing 12 trillion biologically active molecules of thymus protein, and sold in health food stores. If you are fighting an infection such as flu, colds, herpes, shingles, or chronic sinusitis, the recommended dose is one packet every four hours, taken sublingually (dissolved under the tongue). This special thymic protein should help you get back on your feet quickly. Once the symptoms are gone, you can discontinue the treatment.

If you are not sick now but seem to be going from illness to illness, I recommend that you take a maintenance dose of one packet a day indefinitely. This should help you ward off the next infection that comes your way.

Caution: Due to the fact that thymic protein stimulates immune function, it should not be used by individuals with overactive immune systems, such as those with the autoimmune diseases lupus erythematosus and rheumatoid arthritis.

AGE SAVER: Sleep Your Way to a Strong Immune System

Ever notice how, after you miss a few nights' sleep, you seem to catch more colds? That's because T cell production peaks during sleep. If you miss even one night's sleep, a decline in T cells will leave you vulnerable to infection. I cannot overemphasize the importance of a good night's sleep in keeping your immune system functioning optimally.

Keep Exercising

Moderate exercise will also help enhance immune function. As discussed in Step 4, literally hundreds of studies show a positive relationship between moderate exercise and disease. In addition, exercise gets the lymph system, which houses immune cells, moving. Unlike your cardiovascular system, which is powered by the heart, the lymph system has no pump, and its flow depends on bodily movement. Lack of exercise leads to a sluggish system.

You should not overdo exercise, however, because too much of it stresses the immune system. Elite athletes have a higher incidence of infectious diseases than the general population and a much higher rate than moderate exercisers. After a session of strenuous exercise, the production of T cells and other important immune cells slows down. The more intense the exercise, the greater the reduction in these cells. The decline in immune cells persists for one to three hours after exercise. In addition, the production of stress hormones increases with exercise, and as we've seen, stress hormones inhibit immune function. Now bear in mind that I'm talking about *very* strenuous exercise. The Age Loss Program's workout routine is highly effective because it is not too taxing and will benefit you in many ways, including the strengthening of your immune system. Exercise regularly and moderately. If you're a bit under the weather, put off exercise for a day or two.

Maintaining the youthful vigor of your immune system will help prevent most of the problems that have come to be considered a normal part of the aging process. Every step of the Age Loss Program will help maintain the vitality of your immune system. Living an immune-friendly lifestyle—from eating the right food to getting enough sleep and exercise—is the best thing you can do to preserve your health.

There are some people, however, who already have medical problems when they start my Age Loss Program. This stands in the way of their successfully completing the program. Step 10 will help these folks get back on track so that they, too, can *shed ten years in ten weeks.*

Step 10

⁊

REGAIN A DECADE'S WORTH OF HEALTH BY CORRECTING THE GLITCHES

A Special Rx for:

Arthritis

Depression

Diabetes

Gastrointestinal Disorders

Heart Disease

High Blood Pressure

Osteoporosis

Vision Problems

As YOU KNOW, RULE number 1 of my Age Loss Program is that it is never too late and you're never too old to do something positive for yourself. *Shed Ten Years in Ten Weeks* is for everybody, regardless of age or health. Every step of the Age Loss Program will not only rejuvenate the body but also prevent and in some cases even reverse common health problems. Although I firmly believe that you are never too sick to reclaim your health, I also acknowledge that many people already have preexisting medical conditions that may make it more difficult for them to achieve the goals of the Age Loss Program. For those of you who do, Step 10 provides additional suggestions that I generally prescribe or recommend for eight common medical problems. These can be followed along with the basic Age Loss Program. I do not want to imply that I can treat you long distance. My goal is to encourage you to find a doctor who will work with you to incorporate these natural remedies into your life. If you have a health problem, particularly if you are taking any medication, you should be under a doctor's supervision. Although many of the supplements that I recommend may reduce or even eliminate the need for prescription medication, do not discontinue your medication on your own. Always work with your doctor.

ARTHRITIS

Fifty million Americans suffer from some form of arthritis, a disease characterized by the inflammation or destruction of cartilage, a gel-like substance that consists primarily of water. Cartilage has two main jobs: By lining the joints it prevents the bone endings from rubbing together, and it absorbs shock from weight-bearing activities such as walking. Osteoarthritis, also known as "wear and tear" arthritis, is the most common form of this disease, and an astonishing 80 percent of people over fifty suffer from it. Symptoms of osteoarthritis include morning stiffness, especially in the knees and hips, and joint pain, especially in the fingers.

Until recently it was widely believed that once destroyed, cartilage could not be replaced, and therefore the only treatment for arthritis was strong anti-inflammatory medication to mask the pain. We now know that this logic is faulty. There are two natural supplements that stimulate the production of new cartilage. In addition, the anti-inflammatory drugs routinely prescribed for arthritis are notorious for irritating the lining of the stomach, which can cause chronic stomach upset and even gastrointestinal bleeding. Worse, studies suggest that these drugs may actually contribute to the further deterioration of cartilage! I do not prescribe them for my patients; instead I use natural remedies that both control the pain and halt—and sometimes even reverse—the arthritic process.

If you have osteoarthritis, here are some additional supplements you can add to the Age Loss Program's supplement plan.

Glucosamine

Glucosamine is a natural constituent of cartilage that stimulates the production of connective tissue in the body. As people age they are unable to make enough glucosamine, which results in the inability of cartilage to retain water and act as a shock absorber. Several studies have shown that glucosamine supplements not only can relieve the pain of arthritis but even halt the progress of the disease in many people. Anti-inflammatory medications work faster than glucosamine, but over time, glucosamine is more effective primarily because the effect of anti-inflamatory medications can wear off quickly, whereas glucosamine continues to work. Glucosamine gradually tackles the underlying cause of arthritis by restoring lost cartilage. Within two weeks to a month, most people taking glucosamine will feel significant relief. Better yet, glucosamine is safe, and there are virtually no side effects. For those of you suffering from osteoarthritis, I recommend taking 500 milligrams three times daily of glucosamine. In rare instances glucosamine may cause nausea or heartburn, but this can usually be alleviated by taking it with meals.

245

Once you have become pain free, you can reduce your dose to 500 milligrams daily. You can continue taking the glucosamine as long as you need it.

Chondroitin

Similar to glucosamine, chondroitin is also found in cartilage. Studies have shown that chondroitin supplements can reduce the pain of arthritis, and in combination with glucosamine, appear to stimulate the production of new cartilage. Along with glucosamine, I recommend that you take 200 to 1,000 milligrams of chondroitin daily as symptoms warrant.

Capsaicin Ointment

To relieve pain from arthritis, I recommend capsaicin ointment. Capsaicin is a compound extracted from the pepper plant. When rubbed on the skin, capsaicin ointment can relieve the pain and stiffness of arthritis. Capsaicin causes a mild stinging sensation; this in turn triggers the production of a neurotransmitter called substance P, which is involved in sending pain signals to the brain. Repeated applications of capsaicin deplete your supply of substance P and dampen the pain response. Rub a small amount of capsaicin ointment on the skin directly on affected joints (never on irritated skin or an open wound). Within two to four weeks your pain will lessen or be eliminated altogether. Use as needed.

DEPRESSION

More than 17 million Americans have some form of depression at some time in their lives. Depression can be triggered by an upsetting event—death in the family or the loss of a job

—or it can be caused by chemical imbalances in the body, or sometimes a combination of both. I don't want to suggest that a problem as serious as depression should be self-diagnosed or treated with supplements alone. If you are depressed, you need to be under the supervision of a mental health professional or physician who can help design a treatment program. Everyone feels down from time to time, so how do you know if you are really depressed? Symptoms such as a change in appetite or sleep patterns, fatigue, feelings of sadness, hopelessness, or guilt, inability to think clearly or concentrate, or recurrent thoughts of death and suicide are all signs of true depression. If you experience any of these symptoms for two weeks or longer, you should definitely seek professional help. If you don't have these precise symptoms but find you are so sad or distressed that you are unable to function normally, you should still get professional help.

Here are some supplements that I routinely prescribe for patients who have signs of depression. I have found them to be very effective. If you have a problem with depression, talk to your doctor about incorporating these supplements into your treatment plan.

Saint-John's-Wort

Saint-John's-wort, a veritable cure for mild depression, is fast becoming one of the most popular and best-selling herbs in the United States.

Widely used in Europe but newly discovered here, Saint-John's-wort is an especially effective treatment for mild depression. A recent article in the *British Medical Journal* that reviewed more than thirty studies concluded that Saint-John's-wort was as effective an antidepressant as many stronger prescription medications and without some of the unpleasant side effects, including dry mouth, dizziness, and constipation.

Until recently it was believed that Saint-John's-wort was similar in function to a class of antidepressant drugs called monoamine oxidase inhibitors (MAO inhibitors). People who took Saint-John's-wort were advised to avoid foods rich in tyramine, including wine, cheese, and beans, which could interact with MAO inhibitors. The latest studies show that Saint-John's-wort is not an MAO inhibitor, so the good news is that you can eat whatever you like. If you take Saint-John's-wort, however, you must avoid direct exposure to the sun since this herb makes you more likely to burn.

There are numerous brands of Saint-John's-wort to choose from. Take two 300-milligram capsules of Saint-John's-wort daily for ten weeks, or 20 drops of liquid extract twice daily as long as you need it.

DIABETES

More than 14 million Americans have diabetes, a disease characterized by an excess of sugar in the blood and urine. Type I diabetes, also known as juvenile diabetes, occurs primarily in children and adolescents, and is caused by damage to insulin-producing cells in the pancreas. People with Type I diabetes must take supplemental insulin throughout their lives to control blood sugar.

Type II, or adult-onset diabetes, is the most common type, typically occurring in people over forty. Those with Type II diabetes make enough insulin, but the insulin works less efficiently. Nearly everyone over forty experiences some degree of insulin resistance, and at least 25 percent of all adults will develop a condition serious enough to warrant treatment.

There are numerous prescription medications used to control blood sugar, but the problem is that they all have the potential for adverse side effects, including headaches, infection, and even sexual dysfunction. Many diabetics come to the Whitaker Wellness Institute because they are desperate to get off their medication and live a more normal life. Fortunately, when it comes to diabetes, natural remedies are very effective, and the only side effect is a positive one—you feel healthier.

Since 90 percent of all people with Type II diabetes are obese, shedding the excess pounds is one of the best ways to prevent the disease and is also one of the most effective treatments. Diabetics will probably have to follow a more restrictive diet than the Age Loss Program's food plan, which is why it is important to work with a nutritionally oriented physician. The good news is that in most cases Type II diabetes can be controlled by diet, exercise, and supplements, and even Type I diabetes can be greatly improved by making these positive changes in lifestyle.

Most people with Type II diabetes may also have a condition known as Syndrome X, which is characterized by abdominal obesity, high blood cholesterol, high blood pressure, and very high blood triglycerides. In addition to the fish oil capsules I recommend for high triglycerides (see page 255), the supplements I recommend for diabetes are also excellent for Syndrome X. People with Syndrome X tend to be very sensitive to starchy food, which sends their blood sugar and triglycerides soaring. Eliminating all starchy food from their diet (bread, pasta, potatoes, and so forth) can bring their numbers back to normal range.

Here are additional supplements that I recommend for people with diabetes and/or Syndrome X.

Vanadyl Sulfate

Insulin is responsible for regulating the metabolism of carbohydrate and protein by the body, breaking down these nutrients into a form that can be readily utilized by the cells for energy production. Vanadyl sulfate is a biologically active form of vanadium, a trace mineral very similar in action to the hormone insulin.

Vanadyl sulfate can enhance the action of insulin, thereby preventing a buildup of sugar in the blood. I also believe that it may help prevent a mild case of insulin resistance from worsening. I have also found it very effective in the treatment of diabetes. Vanadyl sulfate may reduce your need for other diabetic medication, but if you are diabetic, do not take vanadyl sulfate unless you are under the supervision of your doctor. For my patients with diabetes, I recommend two 45-milligram capsules or tablets of vanadyl sulfate daily. *Since vanadyl can cause a sharp decline in blood sugar, it is imperative that you be monitored by your doctor.*

Lipoic Acid

As part of your Age Loss ODAs, you are already taking 50 milligrams of lipoic acid, a remarkable antioxidant that also helps control blood sugar. In Europe, lipoic acid is routinely given to diabetics to prevent serious complications such as peripheral neuropathy or nerve damage. If you have diabetes, I recommend that you increase your dose of lipoic acid to 300 milligrams daily, so take two 150-milligram doses daily.

Gymnema Sylvestre

Native to India, this herb has been used by that country's healers for nearly two thousand years. Studies show that gymnema sylvestre lowers blood sugar and may help repair damaged cells in the pancreas. Although it has not been scientifically proven, gymnema is also reputed to reduce the urge to eat sweets, which will help curb the urge for dessert if you are trying to lose weight. Gymnema sylvestre is available in capsules. Diabetics should take two 200-milligram capsules daily.

GASTROINTESTINAL PROBLEMS

Gastrointestinal problems, particularly heartburn and ulcers, are common complaints of people middle-aged and older. In general, the high-fiber, low-fat diet recommended in the Age Loss Program's food plan will help keep your digestive system working well. If problems creep up, there are some wonderful natural over-the-counter treatments that will help reduce your discomfort.

But before I detail some of these remedies, let me tell you about some important medical information you should know about ulcers. It has recently been found that ulcers, which were once believed to be caused by excess stomach acid, are now known to be caused by the bacteria Helicobacter pylori (H. pylori). This means that ulcers can now be cured by a short course of antibiotics, yet a surprisingly high number of doctors ignore this fact and still prescribe antacids to patients with ulcer symptoms. If you have ever been diagnosed with an ulcer or have the telltale burning or abdominal pain, make sure that your doctor tests you for H. pylori. Antacids will only mask the symptoms but will not cure the ulcer.

Many people mistakenly believe that heartburn is always caused by *excess* stomach acid, and they take antacids indiscriminately. But in many cases, particularly if you are over sixty, you may have just the opposite problem—you may not have *enough* stomach acid. Instead of taking antacids, you may need to take supplements of hydrochloric acid (HCL). If you suffer from the usual heartburn symptoms, go to a knowledgeable doctor who can give you an accurate diagnosis and the proper treatment.

251

Licorice

When Westerners think of licorice, we typically think of the sugary candy that contains only traces of the real licorice herb. In China, however, licorice is revered as serious medicine. For more than five thousand years Chinese healers have used licorice to soothe painful ulcers and other gastrointestinal problems. Westerners have been reluctant to use licorice because it can raise blood pressure, but a new form of licorice —deglycyrrhizinated licorice, or DGL—is a soothing, safe treatment that will relieve the pain of ulcers and other GI symptoms without increasing blood pressure. DGL helps build up the protective stomach lining that has been worn down by irritation. It also promotes blood flow to the lining of the intestinal tract, which will promote healing. Recent studies comparing DGL and antacids have shown that licorice works as well as, if not better than, many prescription and over-the-counter medications and that people who use it have fewer recurrences. Unlike antacids, DGL does not cause side effects such as nausea, diarrhea, possible liver damage, and possible impotence. DGL comes in chewable tablets. For best results chew two 380-milligram tablets of DGL twenty minutes before eating.

Peppermint Tea

A cup of peppermint tea after meals can have a calming effect on your digestive symptoms and will quickly relieve gas and heartburn. Peppermint teas are sold in supermarkets and health food stores. Be sure to let the tea bag steep for at least five minutes before drinking it. You can drink peppermint tea as often as you need to.

HEART DISEASE

In most cases heart disease can be controlled and even reversed simply by taking the right supplements, eating a sound diet, and following a sensible exercise routine. Every step of my Age Loss Program will have a positive impact on the health of your heart. However, if you are suffering from a heart condition, in addition to what you are already doing I urge you to take the following supplements that we use at the Whitaker Wellness Institute. All of them are sold over the counter in health food stores and pharmacies.

Co-Q10

I regard Co-Q10 as *the* supplement for a healthy heart. As part of the Age Loss ODAs, you are already taking 60 milligrams of Co-Q10 daily. If you have heart disease, I recommend that you increase the dose to 200 milligrams daily.

L-carnitine

L-carnitine is an amino acid found in the heart, brain, and skeletal muscles. I have used L-carnitine to treat heart disease for more than a decade, and the benefits have been well documented in numerous studies published in the *American Journal of Cardiology* and other medical journals. Studies document that L-carnitine can improve stamina and endurance in heart patients, allowing them to exercise without experiencing angina or chest pain. Since regular exercise is one of the best treatments for heart disease—and pain is the primary reason that heart patients don't exercise—this is a real boon.

L-carnitine can also reduce cholesterol levels, boost levels of good cholesterol, and lower high blood pressure, all of which will help prevent heart disease in the first place.

If you have heart disease, talk to your physician about including L-carnitine in your treatment program. I recommend taking two 500-milligram capsules of L-carnitine daily.

Magnesium

Magnesium, an essential mineral for heart health (and one that is often overlooked), decreases blood pressure and improves the flow of blood to the heart. Magnesium will be found in your multivitamin, but I recommend that heart patients take an additional supplement of 500 milligrams daily, preferably in the evening. It has a soothing effect on the body and will help you wind down for the night. (People with kidney failure should not take magnesium supplements.)

Hawthorn

For more than four centuries this "heart-healthy" herb has been used in Europe to relieve angina (chest pain), and irregular heart beat, and as a tonic to strengthen the heart. Studies have shown that hawthorn extract can dilate the blood vessels to the heart, thereby improving the flow of blood and oxygen. I routinely prescribe one 250-milligram capsule of hawthorn daily to my heart patients.

L-arginine

Recently I have added another supplement to my protocol for heart disease: the amino acid L-arginine. Studies have shown that L-arginine can protect blood vessels from atherosclerosis, or hardening of the arteries. As you may recall, in Step 6 I also recommend L-arginine supplements for men with erection problems, to take prior to having sex to increase blood flow to the penis. To get the full benefit of L-arginine for your heart, however, you need to take it every day. For my patients with heart disease, I prescribe 6 grams of L-arginine daily. It is sold as a powder that can be mixed in water or juice. Take one dose daily.

HIGH BLOOD CHOLESTEROL

Niacin

Many people with heart disease also have high levels of cholesterol, a waxy, fatlike substance found in the blood. Niacin (vitamin B3) is a very effective treatment for reducing blood cholesterol levels. Studies have shown that it works as well as prescription drugs but without some of the more dangerous side effects, including flushing of the skin and itching. I recommend a form of niacin called inositol hexanicotinate, which is effective without causing flushing or other discomfort. Take 500 milligrams of inositol hexanicotinate three times daily with meals. (At very high doses, niacin may cause liver damage, so if you take niacin in any form, you should be under the supervision of a doctor.)

HIGH BLOOD TRIGLYCERIDES

Fish Oil

Triglycerides are a type of fat found in the blood, and until recently they were overlooked as a risk factor for disease. We now know that triglyceride levels should ideally be around 150 and that levels over 200 can increase the risk of heart attack and stroke. Similar to high cholesterol levels, high tri-glyceride levels can be detected through a simple blood test. The omega-3 fatty acids found in fish oil are an excellent remedy for high triglycerides. As part of the Age Loss ODAs, you are already taking two capsules of 1,000 milligrams of softgel fish oil daily. If you are diagnosed with high triglycer-ides, I recommend that you double your dose to 4,000 milli-grams. Take two capsules in the morning and two capsules at night.

HIGH BLOOD PRESSURE

Blood pressure measures the force of blood against the arterial wall as it is pumped throughout the body by the heart. High blood pressure means that your heart is working harder than it should to circulate blood; this can damage the heart, arter-ies, and kidneys. High blood pressure is a leading risk factor for heart attack and stroke, and it is called the silent killer because there are rarely any symptoms. You can have very high pressure and feel absolutely fine, but it is inflicting great damage on your body.

A normal adult blood pressure is 120/80. The first num-ber represents the systolic pressure, the pressure of the blood flow when the heart is beating. The second number represents the diastolic pressure, the pressure of the blood flow when the heart is at rest. A blood pressure reading above 120/80 but below 140/90 is considered borderline high blood pressure. Moderately high blood pressure is defined as 140–160 over 90–104. Severe high blood pressure is 160 and higher over 115 and higher. If you have severe high blood pressure, you must be treated by a doctor, and medication may be required. Any blood pressure over 120/80 should be treated but not necessar-ily with medicine. Typically, medication that lowers high blood pressure has many unpleasant side effects, ranging from excessive fatigue, depression, and even impotence. It is far preferable to treat high blood pressure with a combination of diet, exercise, stress reduction, and supplements, and only when absolutely necessary do I order prescription medication. If you have high blood pressure, add the following foods and supplements to your daily regimen.

Potassium

Potassium, a mineral found in fruits and vegetables, can lower blood pressure as effectively as any medication. If you have high blood pressure, I recommend that you get an additional 500 milligrams of potassium daily by eating more fruit and vegetables. One medium-size piece of fruit such as an apple or an orange contains about 300 milligrams of potassium; a banana contains 560 milligrams of potassium. I prefer that you eat fruit rather than take potassium supplements because in addition to containing potassium, fruit is loaded with fiber, antioxidants, and other helpful phytochemicals that can keep you healthy. To obtain 500 milligrams of potassium you will need to eat five or six servings of fruit instead of the three or four I recommended as part of the Age Loss Program's food plan.

If your blood pressure is particularly high, talk to your doctor about changing your diet. When I encounter patients with very high blood pressure, I often put them on a very restricted but potassium-rich diet consisting of brown rice, fruit, and vegetables for two weeks. This diet produces dramatic results, and I have seen high blood pressure return to normal in no time.

Garlic

Healers have known about garlic's powerful effect on the body for centuries. About two thousand years ago, Hippocrates, known as the father of modern medicine, used garlic fumes to treat uterine cancer. Recently, studies have documented that garlic can lower overall blood pressure, and in particular, can have a dramatic effect on systolic pressure (the top number). In Step 2, I recommended that you eat garlic as often as possible, but if you have high blood pressure, I urge you to eat one or two cloves of fresh garlic *every day,* or take a supplemental equivalent. There are numerous garlic products on the market ranging from dried garlic pills, garlic oil capsules to aged garlic extract capsules. The potency will vary from brand to brand, but the label will tell you the equivalent dose in terms of fresh garlic.

OSTEOPOROSIS

About 25 percent of all women and 15 percent of all men will develop osteoporosis, a condition characterized by the thinning of bone, which leaves it vulnerable to breaks and fractures. Losing some bone is part of the natural aging process—the body's repair mechanisms slow down, and so does the production of new bone—but osteoporosis is the *rapid* loss of bone in which whole areas become worn down, particularly in the vertebrae, hips, and forearms. Regular weight-bearing exercise such as walking and jogging will help keep you strong and maintain bone mass, but there are other things you can do to stem the loss of bone and to stimulate the formation of new bone. Small-boned Caucasian or Asian women, smokers, and heavy drinkers of both sexes are at risk of osteoporosis. If you are at risk or if you already have it, here are some supplements that may help protect your bones and prevent further bone loss.

Hormone Replacement Therapy

For women Because bone formation is dependent on hormones, it is not surprising that osteoporosis is a particular problem for postmenopausal women who are deficient in estrogen and progesterone. Hormone replacement therapy is the treatment of choice for women. Estrogen replacement will help preserve existing bone, and tantalizing evidence suggests that natural progesterone may actually stimulate the growth of new bone. Dr. John R. Lee, a California physician, found that natural progesterone therapy was able to reverse osteoporosis in several of his patients, and some women had an increase in bone density. Natural progesterone is sold over the counter at pharmacies and health food stores. On page 192, I tell you how to use it.

For men Because men are bigger boned to begin with, osteoporosis is not as great a problem for them. Nevertheless, one out of six men will develop osteoporosis, and similar to women, hormone replacement therapy may help prevent the loss of bone.

The primary male hormone is testosterone, and as discussed earlier, about 30 percent of all men over fifty have low testosterone levels. In addition to treatment for lack of energy and low libido, testosterone may help men retain bone. Studies have shown that supplemental testosterone causes an increase in bone density and strengthens the muscles that support the bone, thereby reducing the load on the bone. If you have been diagnosed with osteoporosis, I recommend that you talk to your doctor about testosterone replacement therapy.

Calcium

Calcium is essential for building and maintaining strong bones, and few people get enough of it. The multivitamin that you take daily should contain 1,000 milligrams of calcium. If you are at risk of osteoporosis or have osteoporosis, take an additional 500 milligrams of calcium daily to maintain bone and prevent further bone loss.

VISION PROBLEMS

The two most common age-related vision problems are cataracts and macular degeneration, both of which are prevalent in people over fifty. A cataract is a cloudy or opaque covering that grows over the lens of the eye and can cause partial or total blindness. In some cases, the cataract must be surgically removed to restore vision.

Macular degeneration is caused by the destruction of the macula, the part of the eye responsible for central vision—the kind of vision required for activities such as reading and sewing. It is the leading cause of blindness in older adults. Although there are no cures for either of these problems, the right food and supplements can help prevent them or at least slow down the damage inflicted by these diseases.

Following the Age Loss Program's food plan, which emphasizes vegetables and fruits, will help prevent vision problems. In one recent study published in the *Journal of the American Medical Association*, researchers examined the intake of carotenoids (like beta-carotene and lycopene) and vitamins A, C, and E in 365 people with age-related macular degeneration and 520 people without vision problems. They found that the people least likely to develop macular degeneration were those who had the highest intake of green leafy vegetables, particularly spinach and collard greens. In addition to eating your vegetables, I recommend the following three additional supplements that will help preserve vision.

Bilberry

Bilberry contains potent antioxidants, including anthocyanosides, that protect the tissues of the eye and improve the flow of blood to the eye. In one study conducted on fifty patients with cataracts, bilberry supplements actually stopped the progression of cataracts in 97 percent of the cases. Bilberry capsules are available in health food stores and pharmacies. Look for standardized products with 25 percent anthocyanosides and take 80 milligrams twice a day.

Taurine

Taurine is an amino acid that is concentrated in the retina. As we age, our ability to manufacture taurine declines. To fill this gap, I recommend taking 500 milligrams of taurine daily.

Vitamin C

As part of the Age Loss ODAs, you are already taking 2,500 milligrams of vitamin C daily. If you are developing cataracts or macular degeneration, I recommend that you increase your intake of vitamin C by 500 milligrams, a total of 3,000 milligrams daily. Vitamin C will help protect against ultraviolet-light damage from the sun, which is a major cause of cataracts.

Although Step 10 is for people with special medical needs, I want to stress that this is but one step toward achieving wellness. There are nine other steps in this book that will also do you a world of good. Making positive changes in your lifestyle, as outlined in this book, is essential for restoring health, vigor, and vitality. That is what *Shed Ten Years in Ten Weeks* is all about.

Afterword

Keep Going!

Now that you have completed the Age Loss Program, I know you feel happier, healthier, and more vigorous than you have in years. Your body is sleeker and more toned, liberated from ten years' worth of fat. Your skin is softer and more vibrant. Your mind is sharper and more focused. And you are mentally and physically recharged, bursting with energy, with a new-found enthusiasm for life.

These positive changes are a direct result of the ten-step Age Loss Program and, more specifically, all the good things you are now doing for yourself. You are eating the right food, taking the right supplements, exercising regularly, and controlling the negative impact of stress in your life. By incorporating these simple but powerful changes in your daily routine, you have shed the years and reclaimed your health.

The benefits of the Age Loss Program will last well beyond your ten-week investment: You will reap the benefits for years to come. The Age Loss Program proves that we need not surrender to the forces of aging and that it is within our power to control how well we age and the quality of our lives up to our very last years.

Just because the ten weeks are up does not mean that you have to stop. If you want to maintain all that you have gained for your entire lifetime, you should continue following the program indefinitely.

The message of *Shed Ten Years in Ten Weeks* is a life-affirming one; that it is possible to age well in a youthful body and to maintain a strong, active body and mind well into "old" age. The Age Loss Program is your blueprint for a long, happy, and healthy life.

Julian Whitaker, M.D.
Newport Beach, California
August 1997

Resources

The following companies or organizations will provide information on products and services mentioned in this book.

Dr. Whitaker's books are sold in bookstores, health food stores, or by mail order from the Whitaker Wellness Institute Medical Clinic, Inc. The telephone number is 1-800-826-1550.

For information on Dr. Whitaker's monthly newsletter, *Health and Healing*, call 1-800-539-8219.

SUPPLEMENTS AND SKIN CARE PRODUCTS

Forward, Dr. Whitaker's supplement regimen, and the other supplements listed in this book, are available from Healthy Direction, Inc. Call 1-800-722-8008.

FLAXSEED OIL

At the Whitaker Wellness Institute we use flaxseed oil products from these two companies:

> *Omega Nutrition*—Call 1-800-661-3529.
> *Barleans's*— Call 1-800-445-3529.

ORGANIC POULTRY

Call Trader Joes at 1-800-746-7857 to locate a store near you.

SOY FOODS

For information on soy foods and how to use them, call United Soybean Board Hotline at 1-800-TALK-SOY

HIGH-PERFORMANCE HYGIENE

For information or to place an order, call 888-334-8900.

FULL-SPECTRUM LIGHT

To order by mail call Seventh Generation at 1-800-456-1177.

NATURAL HORMONES

For information, call the following compounding pharmacies:

>   California Pharmacy and Compounding Center
>   1-800-575-7776
>   College Pharmacy
>   1-800-888-9358
>   Women's International Pharmacy
>   1-800-279-5708
>   Wellness Health and Pharmaceuticals
>   1-800-227-2627

Dr. Julian Whitaker is the founder of Whitaker Wellness Institute Medical Clinic, Inc., in Newport Beach, California. This full-service clinic, staffed by four doctors and other medical professionals, combines the best of traditional medicine with cutting-edge nutritional and complementary approaches. In addition to individual appointments and two-day intensive evaluations, the Institute offers a one-week residence program of medical testing and evaluation, education and implementation of the basics of the Age Loss Program. For more information on the Whitaker Wellness Institute Medical Clinic, call 1-800-826-1550 or 714-851-1550.

Selected
Bibliography

Abraham, A.S., et al. "The Effects of Chromium Supplementation on Serum Glucose and Lipid in Patients with and Without Non-Insulin-Dependent Diabetes." *Metabolism* 41, no. 7 (July 1992).

Adlercreutz, H. "Lignans and Phytoestrogens: Possible Preventive Role in Cancers." *Frontiers in Gastrointestinal Research* 14 (1988): 165–76.

Adlercreutz, H., et al. "Plasma Concentrations of Phyto-estrogens in Japanese Men." *The Lancet* 342 (November 23, 1993): 1209–10.

Ahlborg, B., et al. "Effect of Potassium-Magnesium Aspartate on the Capacity for Prolonged Exercise in Man." *Acta Physiol. Scand.* 74 (1968): 238–45.

Altura, B., et al. "Magnesium: Growing in Clinical Importance." *Patient Care* (January 15, 1994): 130–50.

Anderson, J. W., et al. "Dietary Fiber and Diabetes: A Comprehensive Review and Practical Application." *Journal of the American Dietetic Association* 87, no. 9 (1987): 1189–97.

Anderson, R. A. "Chromium, Glucose Tolerance, and Diabetes." *Biological Trace Element Research* 32 (1992): 19–24.

Baggio, E. R., et al. "Italian Multicenter Study on the Safety and Efficacy of Coenzyme Q10 as an Adjunctive Therapy in Heart Failure" (interim analysis). *Clinical Investigator* 71:S (1993): 145–49.

Barnes, S., et al. "Soybeans Inhibit Mammary Tumors in Models of Breast Cancer." *Mutagens and Carcinogens in Diet* (1990): 239–53.

Barrett-Connor, et al. "A Prospective Study of Dehydroepiandrosterone Sulfate, Mortality, and Cardiovascular Disease." *New England Journal of Medicine* 315, no. 24 (April 11, 1986): 1519–24.

Batmanghelidj, F. *Your Body's Many Cries for Water.* Falls Church, Va.: Global Health Solutions, 1992.

Bielski, R. J., et al. "Phototherapy with Broad Spectrum White Fluorescent Light: A Comparative Study." *Psychiatry Research* 43, no. 2 (August 1992): 167–75.

Blumenthal, Mark. "Echinacea Highlighted as Cold and Flu Remedy." *Herbalgram* 29 (1993): 8–9.

Burger, H., et al. "Effect of Combined Implants of Oestradiol and Testosterone on Libido in Postmenopausal Women." *British Medical Journal* 294 (April 11, 1987): 936–37.

Carroll, K. K. "Review of Clinical Studies on Cholesterol-Lowering Response to Soy Protein." *Journal of the American Dietetic Association* 31 (1978): 820–27.

Carughi, A., et al. "Effect of Environmental Enrichment During Nutritional Rehabilitation on Body Growth, Blood Parameters, and Cerebral Cortical Development of Rats." *Journal of Nutrition* 119, no. 12 (1989): 2005–16.

Cassidy, A., et al. "Biological Effects of a Diet of Soy Protein Rich in Isoflavones on the Menstrual Cycle of Premenopausal Women." *American Journal of Clinical Nutrition* 60 (1994): 333–40.

Castleman, M. "Red Pepper Is Hot." *Medical Selfcare* (September–October 1989).

Champlault, G., et al. "A Double Blind Trial of an Extract of the Plant Serenoa Repens in Benign Prostatic Hyperplasia." *British Journal of Clinical Pharmacology* 18 (1984): 461–62.

Chandra, R. K. "Graying of the Immune System: Can Nutrient Supplements Improve Immunity in the Elderly?" *Journal of the American Medical Association* 277, no. 17 (May 7, 1997): 1398–99.

"Chronic Stress Is Directly Linked to Premature Aging of the Brain." *National Institute on Aging, Research Bulletin* (October 1991).

Clark, L. C., et al. "Effects of Selenium Supplementation for Cancer

Prevention in Patients with Carcinoma of the Skin." *Journal of the American Medical Association* 276, no. 24 (December 25, 1997): 1957–63.

Cononie, C., et al. "Seven Consecutive Days of Exercise Lowers Plasma Insulin Responses to an Oral Glucose Challenge in Sedentary Elderly." *Journal of the American Geriatrics Society* 42 (1994): 394–98.

Costa, P. T., Jr., et al. "Psychological Research in the Baltimore Longitudinal Study of Aging." *Gerontology* 26 (May-June 1993): 138–41.

Crimi, A., et al. "Extract of Serenoa Repens for the Treatment of the Functional Disturbances of Prostate Hypertrophy." *Med Praxis* 4 (1983): 47–51.

Crook, T. H., et al. "Effects of Phosphatidylserine in Age-Associated Memory Impairment." *Neurology* 41 (1991): 644–49.

Debusk, R., et al. "Training Effects of Long Versus Short Bouts of Exercise in Healthy Subjects." *American Journal of Cardiology* 65 (April 15, 1990): 1010–13.

Diamond, M. C., et al. "Plasticity in the 904-Day-Old Male Rat Cerebral Cortex." *Experimental Neurology* 87, no. 2 (February 1985): 309–17.

Ditre, M. Cherie, et al. "Effects of a-Hydroxy Acids on Photoaged Skin: A Pilot Clinical, Histologic, and Ultrasound Study." *Journal of the American Academy of Dermatology* 34, no. 2, Part 1 (February): 187–95.

Dorgan, J. F., et al. "Antioxidant Micronutrients in Cancer Prevention." *Nutrition and Cancer* 5, no. 1 (February 1991): 43–50.

Dragsted, L. O., et al. "Cancer Protective Factors in Fruits and Vegetables: Biochemical and Biological Background." *Pharmacology and Toxicology* 72, no. 1, Supplement (1993): 116s-35.

Dustman, R., et al. "Aerobic Exercise Training and Improved Neuropsychological Function of Older Individuals." *Neurobiology of Aging* (1984): 35–42.

Earnest, C. P. "The Effect of Creatine Monohydrate Ingestion on Anaerobic Power Indices, Muscular Strength and Body Composition." *Acta Physiol Scand* 153 (1995): 207–9.

Feldman, E. B., et al. "Ascorbic Acid Supplements and Blood Pressure: A Four-Week Pilot Program." *Ann. N.Y. Academy of Science* 669 (September 30, 1992): 342–44.

"Flax Facts." *Journal of the National Cancer Institute* 83, no. 15 (September 7, 1991): 1050–52.

Flood, J. F., et al. "Memory Enhancing Effects in Male Mice of Pregnenolone and Steroids Metabolism Derived from It." *Proc. Nat. Acad. Sci. USA* 89 (1992): 1567–71.

Follingstad, A. H. "Estriol, the Forgotten Estrogen?" *Journal of the American Medical Association* 239, no. 1 (January 2, 1978): 29–30.

Food and Nutrition Research Briefs. Agriculture Research Service, January-March 1993.

Fotsis, T., et al. "Genistein, a Dietary Derived Inhibitor of In Vitro Angiogenesis." *Proceedings of the National Academy of Sciences* 90 (April 1993): 2690–94.

Fulder, S., et al. *Garlic: Nature's Original Remedy.* Rochester, Vt.: Healing Arts Press, 1991.

Gao, Y. T., et al. "Reduced Risk of Esophageal Cancer Associated with Green Tea Consumption." *Journal of the National Cancer Institute* 86, no. 11 (June 1, 1994): 855–58.

Gillman, M. A., et al. "Protective Effects of Fruits and Vegetables on the Development of Stroke in Men." *Journal of the American Medical Association* 273, no. 14 (April 1995): 1113–17.

Giovannucci, E., et al. "A Prospective Study of Dietary Fat and Risk of Prostate Cancer." *Journal of the National Cancer Institute* 85, no. 19 (October 1993): 1571–78.

Gupta, J. S., et al. "Effect of Potassium-Magnesium Aspartate on Endurance Work in Man." *Indian Journal of Experimental Biology* 11 (September 1993): 392–94.

Hargrove, J. T., et al. "Menopausal Hormone Replacement Therapy with Continuous Daily Oral Micronized Estradiol and Progesterone." *Obstetrics and Gynecology* 73 (1989): 606–12.

Hashim, S., et al. "Modulatory Effects of Essential Oils on the Formation of DNA Adduct by Aflatoxin B1 In Vitro." *Nutrition and Cancer* 21, no. 2 (1994): 170–75.

Herve, A., et al. "Effect of Two Doses of Ginkgo Biloba Extract (EGB 761) on the Dual-Coding Test in Elderly Subjects." *Clinical Therapeutics* 15, no. 3 (1993): 549–58.

Heseker, H., et al. "Psychological Disorders as Early Symptoms of Mild-to-Moderate Vitamin Deficiency." *Annals of the New York Academy of Sciences* 669 (September 30, 1992): 352–57.

Hilton, E., et al. "Ingestion of Yogurt Containing Lactobacillus Acidophilus as a Prophylaxis for Candidal Vaginitis." *Annals of Internal Medicine* 115, no. 5 (1992) 353–57.

Hughes, C. L. "Phytochemical Mimicry of Reproductive Hormones and Modulation of Herbivore Fertility by Phytoestrogens." *Environmental Health Perspectives* 78 (1988): 171–75.

Jacques, P. F., et al. "Effects of Vitamin C on High-Density Lipoprotein Cholesterol and Blood Pressure." *Journal of the American College of Nutrition* 11, no. 2 (1992): 139–44.

Jain, A. R., et al. "Can Garlic Reduce Levels of Serum Lipids? A Controlled Clinical Study." *American Journal of Medicine* 94 (1993): 139–44.

Joosten, E., et al. "Metabolic Evidence That Deficiencies of Vitamin B-12 (Cobalamin), Folate, and Vitamin B-6 Occur Commonly in Older People." *American Journal of Clinical Nutrition* 58 (1993): 468–76.

Julius, M., et al. "Glutathione and Morbidity in a Community-Based Sample of Elderly." *Journal of Clinical Epidemiology* 47, no. 9 (1994): 1021–26.

Kamen, B. *Hormone Replacement Therapy, Yes or No?* Novato, Calif. Nutrition Encounter, 1993.

Kamikawa, T., et al. "Effects of Coenzyme Q10 on Exercise Tolerance in Chronic Stable Angina Pectoris." *American Journal of Cardiology* 56 (1985): 247–51.

Kang, S., et al. "The Cosmetic Beautifying Effect of Retinol (Vitamin A)." *Society for Investigative Dermatology* 105 (1995): 556.

Kinsella, J. E., et al. "Dietary n-3 Polyunsaturated Fatty Acids and Amelioration of Cardiovascular Disease: Possible Mechanisms." *American Journal of Clinical Nutrition* 28 (1990): 1–18.

Kleijnin, J., et al. "Ginkgo Biloba." *The Lancet* 340 (1992): 1136–39.

Kreider, R. B. "Effects of Ingesting Supplements Designed to Promote Lean Tissue Accretion on Body Composition During Resistance Training." *Internal Journal of Sports Nutrition* 6: 234–46.

Lee, H. P., et al. "Dietary Effects on Breast-Cancer Risk in Singapore." *The Lancet* 337 (May 18, 1991): 1197–1200.

Lee, J. R. "Osteoporosis Reversal: The Role of Progesterone." *International Clinical Nutrition Review* 10 (1990): 384–91.

Lemon, H. M., et al. "Reduced Estriol Excretion in Patients with Breast Cancer Prior to Endocrine Therapy." *Journal of the American Medical Association* 196 (1996): 1128–34.

Leviton, R. *Brain Builders.* West Nyack, N. Y.: Parker Publishing Company, 1995.

Lipkin, R. "Vegemania: Scientists Tout the Health Benefits of Saponins." *Science News* 148 (December 9, 1995): 392–93.

Loike, J. D., et al. "Extracellular Creatine Regulates Creatine Transport in Rat and Human Muscle Cells." *Proc. Natl. Acad. Sci. USA* 85 (February 1988): 807–11.

Longcope, C. "Relationships of Estrogen to Breast Cancer, of Diet to Breast Cancer, and of Diet to Estradiol Metabolism." *Journal of the National Cancer Institute* 82, no. 11 (June 6, 1990).

Mata, P., et al. "Effects of Long-Term Monounsaturated- vs. Polyunsaturated-Enriched Diets on Lipoproteins in Healthy Men and Women." *American Journal of Clinical Nutrition* 55 (1992): 546–50.

McNamee, D. "Limonene Trial in Cancer." *The Lancet* 342 (September 25, 1993): 801.

Messina, M., et al. "The Role of Soy Products in Reducing Risk of Cancer." *Journal of the National Cancer Institute* 83, no. 8 (1991): 541–46.

Meydani, S. N. "Vitamin E." *The Lancet* 435 (January 21, 1995): 170–75.

Meydani, S. N., et al. "Vitamin E Supplementation and In Vivo Immune Response in Healthy Elderly Subjects: A Randomized

Controlled Trial." *Journal of the American Medical Association* 227, no. 17 (May 7, 1997) 1380–85.

Michnovicz, J. J., et al. "Altered Estrogen Metabolism and Excretion in Humans Following Consumption of Indole-3 Carbinol." *Nutrition and Cancer* 16 (1991): 56–66.

Mindus, P., et al. "Piracetam-induced Study on Normally Aging Individuals." *Acta Psychiat. Scand.* 54 (1966): 150–60.

Morales, A. J., et al. "Effect of Replacement Dose of DHEA in Men and Women of Advancing Age." *Journal of Clinical Endocrinology Metabolism* (1994): 1360–67.

Murray, M. T. *The Healing Power of Herbs.* Rocklin, Calif.: Prima Publishing, 1995.

Packer, L. "Protective Role of Vitamin E in Biologic Systems." *American Journal of Clinical Nutrition* 53 (1991): 1050S–55S.

Packer, L., et al. "Alpha-lipoic Acid as a Biological Agent." *Free Radical Biological Medicine* 19 (August 1995): 227–50.

Pederson, R., et al. "Long-Term Effects of Vanadyl Treatment on Streptozotocin-Induced Diabetes in Rats." *Diabetes* 38 (1989): 1390–95.

Pelton, Ross. *Mind Food and Smart Pills.* New York: Doubleday, 1989.

Penn, N. D., et al. "The Effect of Dietary Supplementation with Vitamins A, C, and E on Cell-Mediated Immune Function in Elderly Long-Stay Patients: A Randomized Controlled Trial." *Age and Ageing* 20 (1991): 169–74.

PEPI Trial "Effects of Estrogen or Estrogen/Progestin Regimens on Heart Disease Risk Factors in Postmenopausal Women." *Journal of the American Medical Association* 273 (1995): 199–208.

Phillips, W., et al. "Strength and Muscle Mass Changes in Elderly Men Following Maximal Isokinetic Training." *Gerontology* 42 (1996): 114–20.

Pierpaoli, W., et al. *The Melatonin Miracle.* New York: Simon & Schuster, 1995.

Pincus, G., et al. "Effects of Administered Pregnenolone on Fatiguing Psychomotor Performance." *Aviation Medicine* (April 1944): 98–135.

Pinnell, S. "Regulation of Collagen Biosynthesis by Ascorbic Acid: A Review." *Yale Journal of Biological Medicine* 58 (1985): 553–59.

Pinnell, S., et al. "Induction of Collagen Synthesis by Ascorbic Acid: A Possible Mechanism." *Archives of Dermatology* (1987): 1684–86.

Press, R. J., et al. "The Effect of Chromium Picolinate on Serum Cholesterol and Apolipoprotein Fractions on Human Subjects." *Western Journal of Medicine* 152, no. 1 (January 1990).

Prior, J. C. "Progesterone as a Bone-Tropic Hormone." *Endocrine Reviews* 11 (1990): 386–98.

Rall, L., et al. "Vitamin B-6 and Immune Competence." *Nutrition Reviews* 51, no. 8 (1993): 217–25.

Rauscher, F. H., et al. "Music and Spatial Task Performance." *Nature* 365 (1993): 611.

Regelson, W., and Colman, C. *The Superhormone Promise.* New York: Simon & Schuster, 1996.

Regelson, W., et al. "Dehydroepiandrosterone (DHEA)-a Pleiotropic Steroid. How Can One Steroid Do So Much?" In *Advances in Anti-Aging Medicine,* Ronald M. Klatz, ed. Larchmont, N.Y.: Mary Ann Liebert, 1996, pp. 287–317.

Reiter, R. J. "Pineal Melatonin: Cell Biology of Its Synthesis and of Its Physiological Interactions." *Endocrine Review* 12 (1991): 151–80.

Roberts, E. "Pregnenolone—from Selye to Alzheimer and the Model of the Pregnenolone Sulfate Binding Site in the GABA Receptor." *Biochemical Pharmacology* 49 (1995): 1–16.

Roberts, H. J., *Defense Against Alzheimer's Disease.* West Palm Beach, Fl.: Sunshine Sentinal Press, 1995.

Robinson, E., et al. "Estrogen Replacement Therapy and Memory in Older Women." *Journal of the American Medical Association* 42, no. 9 (1994): 919–22.

Roebothan, B. V., et al. "Relationship Between Nutritional Status and Immune Function of Elderly People." *Age and Aging* 23 (1994): 49–53.

Rose, D. P., et al. "Dietary Fiber, Phytoestrogens and Breast Cancer." *Nutrition* 8, no. 1 (January-February 1992): 47–51.

Rosenberg, I. R., et al. "Nutritional Factors in Physical and Cognitive Functions of Elderly People." *American Journal of Clinical Nutrition* 55 (1992): 1237S-43S.

Salmeron, J., et al. "Dietary Fiber, Glycemic Load, and Risk of Non-Insulin-Dependent Diabetes Mellitus in Women." *Journal of the American Medical Association* 227, no. 6 (February 12, 1997): 472–77.

Sand, M., et al. "A Controlled Trial of Selegiline, Alpha Tocopherol, or Both as a Treatment for Alzheimer's Disease." *New England Journal of Medicine* 336, no. 17 (April 24, 1997): 1216–22.

Seddon, J. H., et al. "Dietary Carotenoids, Vitamins A, C, and E, and Advanced Age-Related Macular Degeneration." *Journal of the American Medical Association* 272, no. 18 (1994): 1413–20.

Seddon, J. H., et al. "The Use of Vitamin Supplements and the Risk of Cataract Among U.S. Male Physicians." *American Journal of Public Health* 84, no. 5 (May 1994): 788–92.

Shansugasundaram, E. R. B., et al. "Use of Gymnema Sylvestre Leaf Extract in the Control of Blood Glucose in Insulin-Dependent Diabetes Mellitus." *Journal of Ethnopharmacology* 30 (1990): 281–94.

Sherwin, B. B. "Sex Hormones and Psychological Functioning in Postmenopausal Women." *Experimental Gerontology* (1994): 423–30.

Siani, A., et al. "Increasing the Dietary Potassium Intake Reduces the Need for Antihypertensive Medication." *Annals of Internal Medicine* 115 (1991): 753–59.

Sikora, R., et al. "Ginkgo Biloba Extract in the Therapy of Erectile Dysfunction." *Journal of Urology* 141 (1989): 141–88A.

Simopoulos, A. "Omega-3 Fatty Acids in Health and Disease and in Growth and Development." *American Journal of Clinical Nutrition* 54 (1991): 438–63.

Sperduto, R. H., et al. "The Linxian Cataract Study: Two Nutrition Intervention Trials." *Archives of Ophthalmology* 111 (September 1993): 1246–53.

Stampher, M. C., et al. "Vitamin E Consumption and the Risk of Coronary Disease in Women." *New England Journal of Medicine* 328, no. 20 (1993): 1444–49.

Stephens, N. G., et al. "Randomized Controlled Trial of Vitamin E in Patients with Coronary Disease: Cambridge Heart Antioxidant Study (CHAOS)." *The Lancet* 347 (March 23, 1996): 781–86.

Street, D. G., et al. "Serum Antioxidants and Myocardial Infarction." *Circulation* 90, no. 3 (1994): 1154–61.

Sunderland, T., et al. "Reduced Plasma Dehydroepiandrosterone Concentrations in Alzheimer's Disease." *The Lancet* (September 2, 1989): 570.

Tajima, S., et al. "Ascorbic Acid Preferentially Enhances Type I and III Collagen Gene Transcription in Human Skin Fibroblasts." *Journal of Dermatological Science* 11 (1996): 250–53.

Teel, R. W., et al. "Antimutagenic Effects of Polyphenolic Compounds." *Cancer Letter* 66, no. 2 (September 30, 1992): 107–223.

Tenover, J. S. "Effects of Testosterone Supplementation in the Aging Male." *Journal of Clinical Endocrinology Metabolism* 75 (1992): 1092–98.

"Triglycerides Finally Unmasked as 'Bad Actor' in Coronary Artery Disease Drama, Researchers Say." *News from the American Heart Association* (July 1994).

Tucker, D. M., et al. "Nutrition Status and Brain Function in Aging." *American Journal of Clinical Nutrition* 52 (1990): 93–102.

Urban, R. J., et al. "Testosterone Administration to Elderly Men Increases Skeletal Muscle Strength and Protein Synthesis." *American Journal of Physiology* 269 (November 1995): 820–26.

Utian, W. H. *Managing Your Menopause.* New York: Prentice Hall, 1990.

van Papendorp, D. H., et al. "Biochemical Profile of Osteoporotic Patients on Essential Fatty Acid Supplementation." *Nutrition Research* 15, no. 3 (1995): 325–34.

Van Scott, E. J., et al. "Alpha Hydroxyacids: Therapeutic Potentials." *Canadian Journal of Dermatology* 1, no. 5 (November-December 1989): 108–12.

Varma, S. "Scientific Basis for Medical Therapy of Cataracts by Antioxidants." *American Journal of Clinical Nutrition* 53 (1991): 335S–45S.

Young, R. L. "Androgens in Postmenopausal Therapy?" *Menopause Management* (May 1993): 21–24.

Ziegler, R. "Vegetables, Fruits and Carotenoids and the Risk of Cancer." *American Journal of Clinical Nutrition* 53 (1991): 251S–59S.

Index